BE AT MY SIDE

A Father's Journey Through His Son's Traumatic Brain Injury

Paul and Erica Richard

BE AT MY SIDE
A Father's Journey Through His Son's Traumatic Brain Injury
by Paul and Erica Richard
1. FAM02100 – Family & Relationships – Grief
2. OCC011020 – Body, Mind and Spirit – Healing, Prayer and Spiritual
3. SEL021000 – Self-help – Inspirational
ISBN: 979-8-88636-027-1 (paperback)
ISBN: 979-8-88636-028-8 (ebook)

Library of Congress Control Number: 2023908639

Cover design by Lewis Agrell

Printed in the United States of America

Authority Publishing
13389 Folsom Blvd #300-256
Folsom, CA 95630
800-877-1097
www.AuthorityPublishing.com

Preface

This story is being written because we think it can help people. The human brain has a way of fading the bad memories over time, probably so they become more bearable. I could not have recalled all these details without my journal that was kept from almost day one. When the tragedy first struck, my wife Erica told me to journal as I sat there alone and isolated with Dylan in his deep, medically induced coma. Emotions were so high and so raw that I was literally in a stupor for months, arguably years. This journal helped then by allowing me to focus my thoughts and let out my emotions in a more conducive manner. It helps now to recall the feelings and thoughts I went through during this experience. It just isn't possible to remember things accurately with the intense number of emotions and enormous amount of stress I was under. The invasion of COVID-19 took a terrible situation and made it much worse. Around March of that same year, 2020, a pandemic of epic proportions took hold of the entire world. It was like something our generation had never seen and could never fathom…until it hit. It caused widespread panic, seclusion, and for so many, utter hopelessness. It affected the global economy, infrastructure, the demise of many previously successful small businesses, health care systems, and our overall social existence as we knew it. It forced a condition of isolation for me and made me deal with many of my thoughts and emotions alone. Someone once told me, "Your mind is like a bad neighborhood. You shouldn't go there alone," which is an analogy I now understand better than ever before.

I write this now as best my memory can recall, aided by the journal. It is comprised almost entirely from **my** perspective, **my** memory, and **my** notes with Erica helping me organize my thoughts into words. Of course, this journey was different for everyone involved—Dylan's mom, step-parents, siblings, grandparents, and friends. I am not proud of some of my moments along this journey. I cannot guarantee this book is one hundred percent accurate as far as the medical information, but it is one hundred percent true…and we all wish it never happened.

Chapter 1

THE NIGHT EVERYTHING CHANGED

The ominous feeling from that first call will likely never go away; my only real hope is that it fades enough over time that it does not badger me every single day. The sound of the phone ringing never caused me such fear before May 12, 2020. To this day it shakes me to my core if I am sleeping and the phone rings. "Dad it's bad, you have to get to UC Davis Hospital as fast as you can!"

It was about 10:45 p.m. and my wife, Erica, and I were fast asleep, probably for at least an hour. We had both been battling a bit of a cold, so we had taken a dose of NyQuil before bed. This made it even harder to snap out of our sleepy fog and concentrate on the call that was about to change life as we knew it. It was a Tuesday and we both had work to do the next day. Due to the recent COVID-19 pandemic, we were going to be doing all that work from home. I believe the pandemic restrictions had a lot to do with me receiving that phone call in the first place. It was a late spring Tuesday night, and Dylan, then seventeen, should have been wrapping up his senior year at Folsom High School. Perhaps he would have been studying for a final, completing a project, or at least getting up early for school the next day. Dylan was my third child to graduate from Folsom High, so I was aware of the routine. Dylan got by academically but was not a real go-getter with the books; he concentrated his energies on football and friends. We would mostly only see him at mealtime and bedtime because he was busy with one or the other. He had also just competed in the Mr. Folsom High fundraiser, which was sort of a talent show/beauty pageant for young men that the Folsom High School seniors put on every year to raise funds for charity. Dylan was one of those larger-than-life personalities who loved to laugh and entertain. He was the type of person who would run through a brick wall for a friend or a family member. Dylan's older brother, Matthew, the person on the other end of the PTSD-causing phone call, competed in Mr. Folsom High seven years earlier.

I was trying to shake the cobwebs out of my mind and focus on what Matthew was saying. I recall yelling, "What? What is going on?"

The panic in Matthew's voice was pulsating out of the phone. "It's Dylan. It's bad."

The parent/police officer in me kicked in a little bit now, and in a stern voice I recall saying, "Alright Matthew calm down, now tell me what happened." What occurred next has caused me much regret. I am not proud of what my initial reaction was. Matthew told me it was a longboarding accident, and my first reaction was to scold Matthew for longboarding. You see, I knew Matthew owned one, he had told me how he would ride down hills wearing special gloves and make sharp serpentine turns back and forth, a lot like snowboarding. I also knew Dylan borrowed it from time to time. Matthew was a very good snowboarder, surfer, scuba diver, and all-around athlete. Dylan was also surprisingly athletic for his build. Dylan was 5'11" and weighed 220 pounds at the time. I am certain of his measurements because he was in the college football recruiting process and had attended an Under Armor recruit camp where he was accurately weighed and measured to share with college football coaches.

Dylan had played on championship football teams his entire life. I remember one time when Dylan was about nine years old, and it was my first year as an assistant coach on his team. In the middle of practice when Dylan was on the sideline, he absentmindedly held my hand. Nine-year-old Dylan would never have done such a display of affection in front of his friends. He was just so relaxed and happy that he must not have realized it. The city of Folsom, California, loves football. From the age of eight on, boys get exposed to great coaches and a super supportive community encouraging them. Dylan had eaten that up, it became a dominant part of his life. In high school, Dylan would work out with the team and then again later on his own. In a preseason lifting contest his senior year, he won pound-for-pound the strongest kid on the team. It wasn't just Dylan; I lived his football life with him; really, we all did. It was not just me coaching him, the whole family supported him. There was nothing better than Friday night football games at Prairie City Stadium!

Back to the dreadful phone call, Matthew also possesses both intelligence and assertiveness, so when he cut me off with, "Dad, don't!", I immediately snapped out of my wrongful thoughts. Honestly, those words never should have come out of my mouth, but like many things which were about to go down in our lives, there was no way for me to take it back. There were more important, life-threatening things to focus on.

I suddenly realized that poor Erica was in the background saying, "What, what, what is going on!?" She is trying just as hard to wake up and now she is sensing my tension and only hearing half the conversation at most, because I was up and in the walk-in closet already getting dressed. I hung up with Matthew because nothing else was going to come from that conversation; he told me exactly what I needed to know and needed to do. I didn't have much to share with Erica, other than we need to get to UC Davis Hospital and it was regarding Dylan. I got dressed and she did also. She was being super supportive, telling me it's probably "not that bad" and "everything will be alright," but she had not heard Matthew's voice. I knew it was bad, and it was not just from Matthew's words. I felt it inside. I believe to this day that she instinctively knew it was bad, but she was doing all she could to calm my nerves. In retrospect, I used the think that one of the kids breaking a bone or blowing out a knee would have been horrible. But this injury was next-level, and life for everyone in this family immediately changed forever.

Erica clicked into mother-mode and immediately started to think of things we may need at the hospital. My mind was on determining the fastest way to get there. We decided to leave our children, sixteen-year-old Tyler, and his twelve-year-old sister Annabella, at home. I am sure Erica must have told them what was going on, but I honestly don't remember, as I was not part of that; I was busy getting out the door. UC Davis Hospital was about twenty to twenty-five minutes away from us. It was dark, traffic was light. I am not sure how long it took us to get there, but I do know we arrived immediately after Cindy, Pablo, Matthew, and Gabby.

Dylan's family dynamic is a blended bunch. Cindy and I are divorced and have Matthew, Gabby and Dylan. We are both remarried. Erica and Pablo are step-parents to Dylan. Ty, Bella, Zach, and Josh are step-siblings to Dylan. We live about ten minutes from each other. Dylan would spend time at both of our houses during his senior year of high school. I would say there was never anything other than the normal tensions between us. We all got along. We all went to Dylan's football games, and we were all there to walk him onto the football field for his final home football game a few months earlier. Tragically, that is the picture that the local newspaper would use when they reported his accident.

This initial hospital scene was a mess. Being the height of COVID-19, the hospital, just like the country, was operating on panic-driven, sometimes senseless rules, which very likely no one had completely thought out, because how could you? We were in the trenches of a worldwide pandemic that no one really knew how to navigate. Cindy and Pablo had been granted access to the emergency room where the ambulance had taken Dylan, but the rest of us had been stopped at the door by security. Only two people were allowed inside for each patient, and they were checking those people for COVID symptoms before allowing them in. It didn't really matter since no one could see Dylan at this point anyway. This left Erica, Matthew, Gabby, and me outside the ER doors. Literally, that is where we stood. Each of us wishing with our very souls we could get in there and hold Dylan and tell him he will be ok. We were all hysterically crying. It was cold out, so we were shaking from cold as well as emotion, especially Matthew, who was alternating between sadness, shock, and anger. Matthew had been the first one to get to Dylan after Dylan's friend had run to Cindy's house to tell them about the accident. It's a vision I am sure Matthew will deal with the rest of his life. I vividly recall Matthew sitting on the curb outside the ER doors crying and shaking uncontrollably. I didn't know how to help him, since I couldn't control my own shaking and crying. Gabby was there, the former Folsom High cheerleader and whom at the time, was a US Air Force ROTC cadet at California State University, Sacramento. Anyone who knows this giant blended family, knows if you want something organized, planned, and executed, you go to Gabby. She could always get everyone on board. She even had a silly little thing she would do with Dylan and her younger siblings when left in charge, where she would call herself "Southern Mama" and she would speak with an accent and threaten to wash their mouths out with soap if they didn't do what she said. Dylan always responded very well to "Southern Mama." However, there was nothing Gabby could do here. She held Matthew to help with his shivering, tried to comfort me, and planned things with Erica about what we do next. Mostly she just sat there and cried and shivered with the rest of us... helpless, sitting on the curb outside of the emergency room doors.

Matthew and Gabby began to provide a small recollection of what had happened. Dylan and his two friends, Lucas and Jake, were hanging out at Cindy's house around ten p.m. on a Tuesday night. Unfortunately, there was no school and there were no tests to study for. The boys were bored, and Dylan decided to take the longboard from Cindy's garage and go "bomb" a nearby hill. Dylan was convinced these new generation longboards were near impossible to crash. The exact spot where the crash happened and the specific details surrounding how it went down, I do not know, and that is because I choose not to know. I know Dylan was not wearing a helmet when his head impacted the pavement just behind his left ear, and he was traveling at some speed. I don't feel like there is anything else in those details that I need to know which will aid me in healing. That is what this journey becomes; an exercise in using every bit of self-control and self-power to just move forward. Sometimes by the day, but oftentimes, especially in the beginning, by the minute. I do know that the two young men with Dylan that night did exactly as they needed to. When they saw that Dylan had crashed, one of them immediately started sprinting back to Cindy's house to get help and the other got on the phone with 911 to get the paramedics rolling. How quickly Dylan got help was the only reason he even had a fighting chance that night. Cindy's house was located a short distance from a fire station for the El Dorado County Fire Protection District. These heroes were on the scene in minutes, and Dylan was lucky enough that it was a highly trained and experienced crew who realized the severity of Dylan's head injury. I later learned that in the case of traumatic injury, the paramedics aim to be under ten minutes on scene before getting the patient underway to the hospital. This amazing team had Dylan en route to the hospital in three minutes. Even more importantly, they knew UC Davis Hospital, which was not the closest ER, had a Neurological ICU and so they transported him there immediately. With a "when seconds count" kind of injury like the severe head trauma Dylan suffered, both are huge factors in survival.

There we were, outside the doors of the ER, shivering, crying, dying inside to know what was happening with Dylan. Sure, we could have gone and sat in the car, but no, that was too far away. We all felt we needed to be closer to Dylan. Eventually, Pablo came out of the ER door so that I could go in. After being cleared of COVID symptoms, I met up with Cindy in the waiting area. She basically had no more information than we did, though she may have been slightly warmer. A hospital employee was there gathering background information on Dylan. It was hard for either of us to speak through our sobs, and at this point I really had no idea what was happening. There seemed like there was nothing more I could do in the waiting room, so I again swapped places with Pablo and went outside to be with Erica, Matthew, and Gabby.

Erica had moved the car to a parking spot in front so we could now sit in the running car and wait, at least we were warm. There was just literally nothing to do but cry and pray. We couldn't even pray out loud, because no one could speak without sobbing. It felt like an eternity that we sat in that car, but I am sure it was just a few minutes until Pablo came out of the hospital to trade places with me again. Dylan was just back from his first CT scan, and they agreed to let only Cindy and I in to see him. As soon as I got to the waiting area, they led us into the ER.

I will never forget the room. It was small. It smelled sterile and seemed dark. Dylan had a breathing tube sticking out of his mouth and they told us he was in a medically induced coma. There were several people working on him. Machines were quietly whispering. Everything around his room seemed to be humming. This is the first time we met Dr. Z, who would play a big role in this story. She was a shorter lady; all I could see were her eyes above her mask. She seemed subdued to me, but then again, how is a doctor supposed to act under these circumstances? In a tense situation like this, I tend to be more hands off, fact-gathering; and true to form that is how I acted. I stood to one side with Dr. Z while Cindy asked if she could touch Dylan. Cindy walked over to his left side and grabbed his hand and kissed him. Dylan moved his arm ever so slightly toward her as she held him. Dr. Z immediately dismissed the movement saying he was in this deep coma, so that it was likely just a reflex. Bullshit! I saw it. He knew his mom was there, like any boy would. We clung to that movement and his finite level of awareness for days and weeks to come. Since Cindy was by his side, I touched his feet through the hospital sheet. This was my way of letting him know I was there too. Cindy rubbed his arm, and he moved it a second time. We knew that he knew we were there, no matter how deep his coma, he was aware. Unfortunately, that was it for us for now. Dr. Z said he needed surgery, **immediately**. His brain was swelling due to the impact with the street. I had to quickly sign some documents while Cindy showered Dylan with love. I knew they were saying he needed surgery, but I still had no idea how serious the injury was until I asked Dr. Z if this was "life threatening," and she replied, "yes, definitely." I was so stunned that I didn't tell Erica, or anyone about that, until days later. We all knew it was bad, no need to make it any worse. We were told we were lucky because the head of the neurology department was in the building when Dylan arrived at UC Davis, so Dylan would be getting the best treatment and in record-setting time. I believe Dylan was in surgery within an hour of the accident…an amazing feat.

They told us it would be two to three hours for the surgery, a tough enough wait under normal circumstances, but this was a COVID tragedy. Only two people were allowed in the neurosurgery waiting room, so we had to split up. We decided Cindy and Pablo would be in the waiting room while Erica, Matthew, Gabby, and myself waited in a car in the parking lot. We sat there for a little while crying, praying, and sharing ideas of why we were so sure Dylan would make it through this surgery. Since we had been in such a rush to get to the hospital, none of us were really prepared to sit in the car for several hours. The first priority was a bathroom. We tried to use the restroom in the hospital lobby, but unfortunately, UC Davis Hospital security had been instructed to not allow anyone inside for **any** reason (except for Dylan's two allowed visitors), not even to use the restroom. It was a ridiculous rule, but what can we do? We had at least two to three hours, so why not drive out to a gas station, get a cup of coffee, and use the restroom there? Nope, not in this COVID world. Every gas station was either closed, or the employee would not allow anyone inside the building for any reason. By about the third gas station, I believe Matthew chose to relieve himself near a dumpster on the side of the building, but this was not a good option for the ladies. We decided it was probably best to drive all the way home, get everything we needed, and then get back so we were there by the end of the surgery.

It was probably around one a.m. when we got home, any effects from the NyQuil were long gone. We were all wide awake and kept coming up with reasons why Dylan, of all people, would be "fine" at the end of this. I am sure his recording 111 tackles and being co-defensive MVP of his section championship football team just six months earlier, were among the reasons we shared. We quickly used the bathroom, brewed some coffee, and grabbed a few blankets and pillows. We hurried right back to the hospital. I don't know what Erica said to Ty and Bella about the accident, there was no way I could face them and not burst into tears.

We were back in the UC Davis Hospital parking lot by 2:15 a.m. I started to feel like I should notify my family who still live in Pennsylvania about Dylan's accident. There were other boys there when Dylan got hurt who undoubtedly told their parents and friends. I would hate to have my family find out via social media. My sister Donna was a labor and delivery nurse, and I knew she typically began her shift at 7:00 a.m. East Coast time, so at 2:23 a.m. Pacific time, I called her hoping she was awake. Erica and I stepped out of the car to make the call. I didn't want to upset Gabby and Matthew any more than they already were. We had all settled down from the initial shock, into a worried but waiting mode. There was no way I would let them see me struggle with this call. I knew I had to make the call, but I also knew that my emotions were on a hair-pin trigger, and I had no idea what would come out of my mouth. Donna answered the phone immediately and sounded kind of chipper to me, so at least I knew I didn't wake her. I tried to begin to tell Donna what was going on, but my voice just wouldn't work. Emotions would get the best of me, and I would have to hand the phone to Erica to speak for me. It was still cold out, but I didn't feel it. We were standing at an empty bus stop near the ER doors, and I would say a few words, hand the phone to Erica to complete my sentences, and then compose myself and want the phone back. I could think more clearly than I could speak, as if to say the words made things real; confirming I wouldn't be waking up from a horrible NyQuil-infused nightmare.

Donna helped me out by asking me facts, so I would just have to say yes or no. Letting Donna know, however ugly it was coming out, was somewhat relieving. I guess telling my loved ones was a large part of the stress, however subconscious. I asked Donna for help telling Mom and Dad because they were in Pennsylvania also, and I knew my delivery was anything but reassuring. My parents were in their mid-seventies, and this was going to be hard enough on them. My dad had some lingering health issues and had mustered up all his energy to come to California to visit us and see Dylan play football in the fall of 2019. The game he made it to was on a chilly Northern California night and my dad was going to have to leave at halftime to go warm up. In true Dylan style, right before the half ended, the other team tried to throw a flare to a running back out of the backfield and Dylan read it all the way! He picked it off in a full sprint and headed the other way for a defensive touchdown. My dad was beaming from ear to ear when he left at halftime, as was I!

There was another play that season which accurately displayed Dylan's personality. Folsom's archrival Oak Ridge High School was driving to win the game, late in the fourth quarter. Cindy's family, also all from the East Coast, was in town to see the game. With only seconds left in the game and Oak Ridge deep in Folsom territory, Dylan came up with a jarring sack of the Oak Ridge QB, forcing Oak Ridge to try, and miss, a long field goal and sealing the Folsom win. Dylan just had a knack for that sort of thing. Football is much different than a brain injury, but maybe he can do the same thing here…snatch a victory from the jaws of defeat.

Donna decided it was probably best to wait to tell my mom and dad. She would get out of work at one p.m. and would go tell them in person. I was one hundred percent good with that plan because there was obviously nothing anyone could do anyway, except pray. Next, I sent my brother a text. I am not sure how I knew to text him, but I believe Donna said he would already be awake. Todd is a homicide detective and because of that he keeps strange hours. I could communicate with my brother like men do, short texts, just the facts. I was much better at this since I didn't have to speak the words. We only communicated for a few minutes before he told me he was calling Donna while she drove to work to discuss what to do about Mom and Dad. Due to the age of my parents and the COVID lockdown, everyone was keeping their social distance, so it was a real possibility that someone was going to have to tell them about Dylan's accident while staying six feet away from them; more COVID cruelty. Donna and Todd made the decision to call my mom and tell her. My mom is a retired nurse, she has seen and dealt with tragedy; of course, she would be great at handling this. To this day I don't know who made that call, or how it went, all I know is that a few minutes later my cell phone rang, and it was my mom…**exactly what I didn't want**. I was afraid that hearing my emotions would give the poor woman a heart attack, but as this journey was to show me time and time again, you never really know what is inside someone. My mom was strong and calm on the phone, like Erica and Donna, and even Cindy (the little bit I had seen her), I believe she was in "mom"-mode. There were still times I would get too emotionally choked up to speak, but Erica was there to take the phone and finish the sentence, or the thought. I would always get right back on the phone as soon as I could so my mom would know I was ok. We were still out at the empty bus stop outside the ER doors standing in the cold weather, shivering, and crying, because I didn't want Matthew and Gabby to see me struggle this way. I am supposed to be the strong one. The call with my mom was successful in relieving that stressor for me. Afterwards, I felt better and could go back to focusing on Dylan.

I am a little foggy on times, but I believe it was around four or five a.m. until we were told the surgery was finished. I recall someone saying the surgery took four hours. I switched places with Pablo and took up a spot in the Neuro ICU waiting room. Pablo had exited out of the ER doors to come to the car but when I tried to enter through those doors, the security guard stopped me. COVID rules dictated that you could only enter through the ER doors if your loved one was in the ER. Dylan was now in the Neuro ICU, so I could not enter that way. I had to walk all the way around the outside of the hospital to the main entrance to go inside. Even the simplest things were not easy. Once inside the main entrance, I was directed to two security guards who were at least personable. While they checked to see if I was allowed to enter, one guard asked me if the other one looked like Draymond Green from the Golden State Warriors basketball team. Just asking the question made them both laugh. Not to mention that with a mask on, he really did. You might think this would be bothersome to me given the tragedy that was unfolding around me, but in some strange way it made them seem like real people, and sort of reminded me that Earth was still spinning. They gave me a security sticker and directions to the correct floor. When I got to the third floor, I showed the nurses a picture Cindy had texted me of the waiting room number. Everything was off due to COVID, so even the staff had to search a few rooms until they found it, but at least I was there.

It was only a few minutes until someone came in and briefed us on the surgery. For the life of me I can't recall who oversaw briefing us, or what exactly they said, only that it was a lot of "wait and see and pray." They then took us right in to see Dylan. A much more shocking sight than the ER visit. Dylan's head was shaved and full of stitches, he had a breathing tube down his throat, and he was in a medically induced coma. I remember them saying he may have to be like that for weeks. Weeks? How in the world will I deal with this for weeks?

Chapter 2

THE EARLY ROAD

Now the education began, it was time to learn about severe brain injuries. I remember being offended they used the word *"severe"* and not just a "brain injury." I began learning things I never wanted to know, things I never knew existed and yet were now, extremely important. We had to learn on the fly, because more than I even comprehended then, we would have to fight for everything Dylan needed to survive this. Along with the education, came the waiting. As I said earlier, we were never going to leave Dylan's side. There was no way we were going to allow Dylan to wake up alone in a hospital bed. As it turns out, we had plenty of time for that. Since Dylan was seventeen, about five weeks from his eighteenth birthday at the time of the accident, he was medically considered a pediatric patient, so COVID pediatric rules dictated we could have twenty-four-hour access to him. Had Dylan been five weeks older, they said we would have only had access to him during visiting hours, which is a fight I am glad we avoided. I don't even want to think about what would have happened if we could not be with him. The hospital came up with the plan that only Cindy and I can visit him, and only one of us at a time. Based on that, we decided to split the days into twelve-hour shifts. We had to always wear a mask while in Dylan's room and we were given a hospital chair in the corner for us to sit on. We were told that stimulation was bad for Dylan. The room was kept cold and dark, with little to no light. They said that was best for Dylan at this stage, so we never complained.

Cindy wanted to take the first shift, so I headed out to the car with Erica, Matthew, and Gabby to go home and get some sleep. Erica saw me walking toward the car and thankfully jumped out and met me halfway there because when we embraced, I lost it. She literally held me up and kept me from falling, as my emotions poured out right there in the parking lot. I could not speak or communicate for quite some time. She probably thought Dylan had died. Matthew and Gabby gave me some time before coming out for an update and I was able to pull it together and give them the plan. I am good with facts. We were heading home for some sleep; except maybe for thirty minutes or so before the accident, we had all been up at least thirty-six straight hours.

Lying in bed crying and trying to fall asleep, Erica was by my side comforting me. She had been so strong all day, usually the role I like to fill. The Guardian Angel Prayer kept going through my head.

Angel of God, my guardian dear, to whom his love, commits me here. Ever this day, be at my side, to light and guard, to rule and guide. Amen.

I was raised Catholic and always held my beliefs privately. I was an occasional church goer as an adult; better at sending my kids to CCD classes than going to Mass myself. Since I had met Erica, she had taught me to be more open with all my feelings, including my religious ones. I always felt I lived a life reasonably true to my upbringing and tried to concentrate mostly on family. I shared with Erica that I was thinking of that prayer and to my surprise, she knew it and said it with me. She jumped out of bed and retrieved a book, a Bible I believe, and handed me a laminated card with the Guardian Angel Prayer on it. I fell asleep with the prayer card in my hands, and I carry that card with me to this day. I got about two and half hours of sleep before waking up, but it was long enough to have a dream about Dylan. I was in some kind of a warehouse and had to pick up these big black objects by hand and move them to the other side of the warehouse. The warehouse was giant, and the black objects were endless. The more objects I moved, the better it was for Dylan. I guess this was my brain's way of coming up with something I could physically do to help him.

When I woke, I got up and got dressed. I put that prayer card in my wallet and headed to UC Davis Hospital. I said that prayer, and many others, over Dylan in his hospital bed countless times; I even wrote the prayer in his logbook (a small notebook Cindy and I kept to pass information back and forth), and I shared that prayer with my extended family. I probably learned that prayer when I was seven years old and don't know the last time I recited it, but I recalled it easily, word for word. The only thing which would break up the flow of the prayer was my sobbing, but I would just start over.

The shifts in the hospital in the beginning are a bit of a blur. I remember always being freezing cold, but eventually I learned to wear several layers of clothing to fend off the icy room temperatures. These early shifts were literally minute by minute, not hour to hour, praying for Dylan's survival. The staff at UC Davis was truly amazing. The nurses began to teach me what some of the numbers on the screens meant: the first big hurdle for Dylan was to monitor inter cranial pressure (ICP). Dylan's ICP was the biggest threat to him right now. High pressure in the brain can cause major damage. Therefore, Dylan had the left side of his skull removed the night of the accident, to relieve some of this intense pressure. The brain had some room to swell now, hopefully limiting damage. The nurses had to explain things to me again, and again. Because I was so emotional, I couldn't retain much. All I knew was the ICP had to drop, so that's where I concentrated. Unfortunately, Dylan had always tended to swell a lot from injuries, but I am referencing this from things like ankle and hand injuries. How could I know how his brain would react?

Dylan's ICP numbers were very high the first night. They consistently hovered around twenty. A surgeon came to see Dylan that first morning and told me was almost positive that Dylan would need a second surgery. I really did not want that for him. I sat in his room staring at his ICP number just praying it would go down, even just a little. The nurses worked twelve-hour shifts and switched at seven. Cindy and I decided we would switch at six a.m. and six p.m., so we could be there when the nurses rotated and listen in on their updates to each other. This way we got to be briefed by the nurse whose shift was ending and help to relay information to the on-coming nurse. Someone decided that due to COVID, Cindy and I could not be in the room at the same time, even for a minute, so we had to meet in the lobby each time we switched. We would give a quick briefing and then hurry up to the room to be by Dylan's side. We would text each other when we got to the hospital, then meet in a corner of the lobby so not everyone would see us crying and giving updates. Dylan was a severe case, so the nurse working with him was assigned **ONLY** to him. There were times he even had two full-time nurses, just designated to care for him. Later that morning, with a little tinkering of meds, that inter cranial pressure (ICP) had dropped down to sixteen.

I learned very quickly that Dylan was super sensitive to any stimulation, even something as slight as the automatic blood pressure cuff going off would cause Dylan's ICP number to rise. So started this crazy routine of me sitting in a corner of Dylan's room, the lights dim, the temperature cool, just staring at the ICP display, crying, and praying that the number would go down. Sometimes it clicked down a number and sometimes it went up. I could only sit there, trying to control it through my will and my prayers. I thought things were going ok until around 11:30 (a little over twelve hours since the accident), and they came to take Dylan for a CT scan. I was not allowed to go, so I sat in the chair and waited. Around one p.m. I was told the CT scan looked good and was being sent to surgeons to be analyzed. By two p.m., Dylan was being prepped for surgery to have the right side of his skull removed also. I was texting like crazy, trying to let everyone know he was going back into surgery. I knew everyone wanted to be at the hospital while Dylan was in surgery. Just like we had done the night before.

Dylan's ICP numbers had spiked to twenty due to the stimulation of the CT scan but had generally been holding steady around sixteen. I was told that sixteen was high but it was acceptable given the severity of the injury. So why does he need the second surgery, why right now? I began to argue with the surgeon a little bit. Here I am, less than twenty-four hours into my TBI education and I am questioning the experienced surgeons. If the CT scan spiked his ICP number, then what was the surgery going to do? I was panicking, borderline angry, and all alone. I couldn't even make a phone call from Dylan's room, I could only text people and wait for responses. How am I supposed to know what is right? The surgeon explained that they follow ALL of Dylan's vital numbers, not just the ICP. The CT scan was good, but the doctor meant "good" in that they believed Dylan could **survive** the surgery. They were all convinced he needed the pressure release of having a double craniotomy. It was also explained to me that the two best surgeons were both at the hospital right now, and both would be named on the surgical authorization form. These amazing and experienced surgeons would work together on Dylan. Dylan would have the best medical team UC Davis had to offer to get him through this surgery. If he went in for it **right now.** If we waited and he needed the surgery in the middle of the night, he would have to go with whomever was available. COVID had all hospitals stressed for workers, so this was a real concern. I agreed to the surgery and a flood of people came parading into Dylan's room for my signature; anesthesiology, respiratory, even someone to sign me up for text updates during the surgery. I signed all the authorization forms. I barely got to give Dylan a quick kiss on his cheek before he was wheeled away.

Some confusion followed for me, because no one knew where COVID rules would allow me to sit and wait during the surgery. They first took me down a floor to the pediatric waiting area, which was totally deserted...not even a receptionist. I had to be escorted there and passed through several doors that needed to be opened with a card reader. This was clearly not going to work. We wanted the same set up as the first surgery, and Cindy would never be able to switch with me in this secure, deserted room. I asked if we could use the same waiting area we had the night before, and they agreed. They said they would let the surgeon know which waiting room the family would be in. As soon as Cindy and Pablo got to the hospital, I switched with them so they could be together in the waiting area. I would sit in the car with Erica, Matthew, and Gabby, just like the night before. We all even sat in the same seats, as an unspoken, superstitious commitment.

The text updates did not work very well, as we didn't get enough of them, but we did get one to let us know the surgery had begun. The mood in the car was better than the night before; lighter and a little more upbeat. I still had my truck at the hospital since I had come in earlier. We checked on it and found out I had a parking ticket for being in a spot more than two hours. How stupid is that?! The parking lot was largely empty due to COVID, but they were still giving tickets. Matthew worked on filing an appeal to the ticket, and Erica and I moved my truck to the parking garage. Small distractions like that made the time go by with a little less of the thundering silence, in not yet knowing Dylan's well-being. Matthew, who was in his second year of law school, decided to appeal to the emotions of the parking authority, rather than any legal basis. A wise choice, as they eventually responded that the ticket was dismissed.

After a while, Erica and Gabby needed to use the restroom. This time the hospital let them individually use the lobby bathroom. As we would continue to find out, there was rarely any consistency with the COVID rules. I took the opportunity to speak to Matthew about PTSD. We cried as I explained that I had spoken to a psychiatrist once, after I witnessed a traumatic death while on patrol as a uniformed police officer. I told him it could be useful to speak to a stranger, rather than just speaking to your family. I reassured him that he can speak with me about it anytime but speaking to someone who is trained to listen and to help deal with the feelings, is sometimes even more effective. Of course, as a dad, I was worried about how this was going to affect all my children's lives. I was scared he would keep the feelings inside, like I tend to do, but to my surprise, he called our insurance, Kaiser Permanente, to inquire about speaking to someone. I love how open to ideas he can be.

About halfway through the procedure, we decided to walk to a Starbucks about a half-mile from the hospital. The sitting in silence can be unbearable. We all ordered drinks, plus we got some for Cindy and Pablo. Erica and I were able to meet Pablo in the lobby of the hospital and hand off their drinks. We were not back at the car too long before Cindy texted and said Dylan was out of surgery. Pablo walked out of the hospital and handed me his admission sticker, so I could bypass the check in and get to the waiting area more quickly, to meet up with Cindy. It turns out, even with the sticker swap, I was too late. The surgeon was gone before I got there. Cindy was talking with two nurses when I arrived. Apparently, the surgeon was an older man and had a rough communication style. From what I gathered, all he said to Cindy after the surgery was that it went, "as expected, or better." Her natural question as a mother was to ask if he had to put the electrode back in Dylan's head, because she believed Dylan didn't like it. Probably a silly question from a surgeon's point of view, but as we eventually learn through this journey, if we don't question everything, sometimes things are done incorrectly. The old surgeon's response was to throw his hands in the air and storm away. Cindy was laughing about it with the nurses. They were saying they were all scared of the grumpy old man, but the good thing was they respected his surgical skills. We were told Dylan was being sutured up, which would take two to two and a half hours to complete (yeah, that's a lot of sutures). I left the hospital to bring Erica, Gabby, and Matthew up to speed and gave Pablo his admission sticker back. We decided to go home to get a little sleep. Jay, my boss who lived several hours away in the LA area, had an Olive Garden dinner waiting for us.

I want to take a moment to emphasize, and acknowledge, the support we received from people during this journey. When we say the help was incredible and truly helpful, seems to me, to fall far short of the truth. We are **all** in agreement as one family, for Dylan, that this would have been a very different type of experience and possible ending, were it not for the love, prayers, and general, overwhelming support and encouragement from everyone around us. There is no way we could give all the effort we needed to give to Dylan without that support. This accident completely uprooted our worlds as we knew it. I mean...**<u>obliterated</u>**. Our extended families were a gigantic support. My brother-in-law and sister-in-law, Paul and Lori, brought us a meal that very first day. Both provided emotional support throughout this tragedy. Erica described to me several times when she was emotionally drained and lying on the floor of her closet hiding her crying that she would call her sister for support. It didn't matter time or circumstance; they were always there when needed.

Another big group of support was the Folsom football families. I say the Folsom football families because that is who organized much of it, but the support from football fans came from all over, archrivals, and even strangers. The law enforcement community also came through with a tremendous amount of support. I currently work for a federal law enforcement agency, but it was countless members of the law enforcement community, from all over the country, from various agencies and affiliations, who contributed. I worked for the

Upper Merion Police Department in King of Prussia, Pennsylvania, fifteen years earlier, and they sent support like I had never left. I do not believe we cooked a meal for the next **thirteen weeks.** That is not just at my house, but Cindy's house also, so twice the number of meals. Some people cooked for us, some sent delivery people, and some sent gift cards. Not only were the meals provided, but it was all organized. Jay, and Erica's dear friend Heather, handled the meals for our house. I was so consumed with just trying to get through every day I do not know who coordinated things for Cindy's house. The meals were a tremendous stress relief to me. At the time, I did most of the cooking for my family and it would have been a worry to me in not being sure my family was eating correctly. It was early COVID, the kids were trying to home school, grocery shopping was weird, toilet paper was scarce. I was essentially unavailable for everyone in my family, except Dylan. He took 100 percent of my energy and most of Erica's energy went in to supporting me. Family, friends, and community kept us afloat, and Jay was a giant part of that. It is one of those things as a man you know you will never be able to pay back.

The next morning, I awoke to some texts from Cindy saying Dylan's numbers were great. She said I was lucky I didn't see him after surgery because he was very swollen and weak. However, he rebounded throughout the night and was steadily around an eight ICP now. I drove to UC Davis and Cindy and I met in the lobby for our brief update before I headed to his room. It was much more relaxed in there now. Everyone was calmer. The entire day, I never saw his ICP above thirteen, even when stressed by the blood pressure cuff, or anything else. When I left at six p.m., he was at a nine ICP even though they had slightly reduced some of his meds. Maybe we were through the worst? Right before I left, Dylan let out a slight cough when they were cleaning his breathing tube. The nurse said, "Given the amount of sedation he was on, it's likely a cough reflex," but it was still a good sign! When I arrived home, I gratefully ate a Chick-Fil-A sandwich someone had contributed to our family for tonight's dinner, before going to bed.

Now, starting this night, something changed for me. I have been coping so far with only light over-the-counter medicinal assistance. I am not a big drug person; I have been on cholesterol-lowering medications for years but never anything to cope with stress, or anxiety...even though I have a family history of it. Since Dylan's accident, I had been taking some Tylenol PM to help me sleep, which got me two and a half hours the first night, and maybe six hours the second night. Erica, with a little assistance from my mother, convinced me to speak to my doctor about prescribing something to help "take the edge off." I was not crying all the time, but certain triggers were causing uncontrollable tears. To be honest, it could sometimes interfere with getting facts from doctors. It sounds kind of strange, but it was the acts of kindness from people that sent me into tears more than anything. I was not the person who ever needs that stuff...until now. I really wanted to be able to control the crying a little bit; my eyes were swollen, my nose hurt from wiping it, and deep down I knew I could not control it. I also knew I needed to be able to get some sleep.

Even when it came time to speak with the doctor about getting some help with it, Erica had to assist me. We called the advice line and had to relay to the nurse our recent tragedy. Like previously, during the call I choked up, and Erica had to take over. We were transferred to someone else and had to tell the story again, and **again** I couldn't speak all the words. They wanted to send me to a psychiatric help line, but we refused. I was not suicidal, internally I was strong, I knew I would do everything I needed to. I just couldn't speak my thoughts or feelings without tears consistently flowing out. Finally, they set a phone appointment for me to speak to a doctor the next day. Erica suggested 11:30 a.m. and said she would meet me at the hospital for lunch and help me through the call. I am so thankful that she did! When the call came around, of course I minimized my emotions to the doctor, and he was inclined to not prescribe me anything. Erica took over the call and gave a far more accurate description of what I was going through and even recommended a drug. The doctor agreed and we ate lunch in the car before Erica left, and I headed back in to Dylan. I was scared to even take these lunch breaks, but I had to, as they didn't allow me to eat in Dylan's room. Erica went to pick up the prescription for me, but of course due to COVID, she had to sit in her car for forty-five minutes until someone came out of the pharmacy and delivered the pills to her car. Nothing could be easy. When I got home that night, I went to sleep with my first dose in me and slept straight through to my five a.m. alarm. My first real sleep since the accident. With this twelve-hour shift system, if I was efficient with everything else, I could get seven to eight hours of sleep before getting right back to the hospital, which with traffic, was a thirty-minute drive away.

Waking up from this first "real sleep," I had a few text updates from Cindy and called my mom on the drive to the hospital. As I mentioned before, my mom is on the East Coast and is three hours ahead of us in California, so driving in at 5:30 a.m., is 8:30 a.m. to her. I could give her a morning update on Dylan, and she could be reassured that I was also hanging in there. This time I spoke to her with no tears. I took a half of a pill when I got to the hospital and was way better with the emotions all day long. I really was better able to communicate with doctors, nurses, and family, because I was not always on the verge of tears. We had several text groups set up for updates, so when I sent one text, I would copy it and send it two or three times. I sent A LOT of texts. It is a cold and unemotional way to communicate…but it was all I had. I received a lot of supportive responses, but the effect is greatly diminished over text.

Chapter 3

BRACING FOR THE STORM

MAY 16, 2020 – FOUR DAYS SINCE THE ACCIDENT.

Today I would call another relaxed day. Dylan was given a bath overnight and his numbers have remained good. All the doctors seem pleased, and his sedation is beginning to be lowered. He looks closer to being asleep now, as opposed to the quarter-open "zombie eyes" he had the past few days. The nurse said his cough is strong and he blinks, but he has no gag reflex yet. All these seemingly small things are important milestones that I had no comprehension I would **ever** be thinking about. Under heavy sedation, the gag reflex is often first to go, and last to come back. The drain tube on the left side of his head was removed because it is no longer draining any fluids. This is another good thing!

I do my best to keep my journal filled with mostly positive thoughts, but I must vent about two complaints. Firstly, COVID restrictions—while some of them are necessary—mostly just confuse the families, patients, and hospital staff. To make it even worse, the COVID restrictions are **always** changing. No one knows what they are doing, or **why.** I am at the single lowest point of my life, and hospital administrators are 100 percent convinced that if even ONE more person comes in the room to help me watch Dylan, COVID will be spread. Yes, I said "help me" because I know now that I need it. Dylan needs the prayers, but I need the support.

My second complaint is the hospital, and the ridiculous enforcement of its parking. We are on COVID lockdown, so the parking lots and garages are generally empty. In four days, the hospital has given me two $43 tickets for parking in the wrong areas. I am an educated man and have twenty-eight years in law enforcement experience. Granted, I am under a ton of stress and likely not thinking clearly, but I am trying. And yet somehow, I still can't figure out where to park in a mostly empty parking garage so as not to get a ticket. My son is fighting for his life, but I must put my energy toward parking regulations. It just seems like the hospital would have figured this out by now. There are vending machines to pay for parking, but they have signs saying parking is free. There are some signs about permit parking, but they are small and not well-placed. There are other signs that say temporary parking, which also make little sense. With all this confusion and upheaval, what does the UC Davis system do? They aggressively issue parking citations at a facility under construction and harsh COVID restrictions. I know this is likely just one or two incompetent people within the system with hundreds of brilliant and wonderful health care professionals, but it is something I am dealing with and seems surreal with everything else going on in my life.

The days with Dylan go by slow now, but that's ok. I listen to Dylan's rhythmic breathing and wait for any machine to beep and destroy the rhythm. The ICP number has been staying in good ranges, so I no longer feel the obsessive need to stare at it. Now, I just glance at it occasionally. Any noises coming from his machines for the past twenty-four hours have been for relatively minor issues or patient maintenance, usually empty IV bags and whatnot. Doctors, technicians, and nurses come in and out regularly, but only to glance at things. Of course, they also monitor Dylan remotely. The big action today was the removal of the right-side drain tube and Dylan had a bowel movement! He fought that bowel movement for as long as he could but finally gave in. It's a good sign again. They even had to put wrist restraints on Dylan, because he is getting to the point in the lightening of his meds that he may wake up enough to try to remove his breathing tube.

MAY 17, 2020 – FIVE DAYS SINCE THE ACCIDENT.

I feel like we have turned a corner. Dylan was up to as much as 40 mg of Versed and by the end of the day he should be around 12 mg; that is the heaviest sedation drug he is on, but it is not the only one. He is on so many IVs that it takes two IV trees to hold all the bags. The drug level is dependent upon the amount of swelling and the ICP, but everything is seemingly headed in the right direction. Although, they always warn us that it can change in an instant. The doctors and nurses play this incredible dance between shutting down his brain and allowing him to wake up. At 40 mg of Versed, Dylan is so deeply sedated that the machines breathe for him. Although Dylan is so strong that he sometimes breathes over the machine, causing it to beep. They basically shut the brain off to let it begin to heal. Dylan seems ready to begin to enter the recovery stage. No one knows what that recovery will look like. I pray for the best. I hear men in Dylan's age group respond better to this type of injury than most. The nurses are the most encouraging to us. Today the nurse told me that the male brain continues growing until the age of twenty-four and can remap around damaged areas. This is exactly the kind of thing I need to hear right now. There have now been many encouraging signs, and we have received so much help and encouragement after there being so much doubt. In the end, all I really have is prayer and I hang on the hope that nothing goes south suddenly. I also pray Dylan feels no pain or discomfort as he comes out of this, and I pray we get our old, vibrant, loving Dylan back. Everyone loves this kid. Dylan is supported by two good and loving families, a lot of very good friends, football families, distant relatives from all over the world, and even strangers who send money, well wishes, and prayers. A huge wave of support has formed since the minute he fell. I can only dream that it has the happiest of all endings.

I love you, Dylan! This is day five of sitting by your bed and I will sit here as long as it takes. Take your time in there, do it right. We can see how strong you are on the outside. Show us how strong you are on the inside. Doctors and nurses are constantly commenting on how physically strong you are. You got this!

MAY 18, 2020 – SIX DAYS SINCE THE ACCIDENT.

The days have all just blurred together. The medicine reduction continues. The nurse today is Toby. Toby is an excellent nurse with an Australian accent. He has some sons of his own and is always friendly and upbeat. He is quickly becoming my friend. Toby was nice enough to explain Dylan's care to me in football terms. He said this is the Super Bowl for Dylan's care team. This is the reason these incredible people do what they do. They have the chance here to save the life of a thriving seventeen-year-old young man. Many patients who come into this neurological intensive care unit are on the back end of their lives and the focus becomes comfort and quality of life. With Dylan, this care team can make a difference which will last a lifetime. Of course, I loved his description of his motivation. Toby also gave Dylan a tennis ball to hold. Dylan seems to subconsciously hold the ball most of the time.

Toby said it is up to the doctors on how quickly they reduce the Versed, but everyone wants Dylan off it. There are too many bad side effects to Versed. Dr. M told me today that he thinks Dylan may be off Versed in the next one and a half days at this rate. Dylan is at 12 mg now and will be reduced by 1 mg every three hours. It is a slow process, and it is tough for me, because I see his ICP numbers begin to rise but the doctors are confident about their process. Mostly, they are confident because they know they can increase the Versed if ever they need to. They are pushing for the reduction but that's because they feel that is best for Dylan.

I am doing alright today. I am a little more emotional than I was the last two days, but still ok. Today I heard from Coach Daberkow, who is the head coach at Concordia University in Nebraska. This is one of the schools that offered Dylan a football scholarship and one in which I visited along with Dylan back in January. Coach Daberkow told me he is praying for Dylan. I also recently heard from Coach Regalado from Clarke University, in Iowa, where we also visited in January. He told me he is not only praying for Dylan, but his scholarship is open for him when he is recovered, with or without football. That got me crying a little, but who could help it? The morning of Wednesday, May 13, Dylan and I were supposed to have a phone call with Coach Pukszyn, the head football coach at Moravian University, and some admissions people. Moravian University is my alma mater. I really thought Dylan was going to end up playing there, on the same fields where I played, so many years ago. Now that seems insignificant. I also just found out that Matthew broke up with his long-time girlfriend. I worry about the impact that may have on him, as he already is dealing with so much.

I guess I was naive and expected the reducing medication days to be easier. Things are still very tense, as I am always watching the numbers and always worried that he is not responding in the right way. I know I must stop with micro-analyzing every beep and every number, but I can't. Relaxing is the hardest thing to do during this ordeal. I am constantly on edge that something will go wrong. That tension is exhausting. I sleep, but it is not restful. I sleep like I am in a hurry to wake up and get back to Dylan's side, even though there is nothing I can do when I am by his bedside except stare at the machines and worry. I am stuck! Where do I go? What do I do? Every day is just like the day before. Its's like some terrible Groundhog Day effect. Erica has been wonderful, but it is still just so weird, our roles changed on a dime and all she does now is try to support me. I want this to change, but only if it is good change; if I can't have that yet, then I will stay right here with this.

MAY 19, 2020 – SEVEN DAYS SINCE THE ACCIDENT.

We were cruising right along this recovery path and then I woke up this morning to BAM! Dylan has a fever. I thought we were on our way out of this. Why can't I just get a break?! I allowed myself a glass of wine last night before bed, and things were feeling upbeat. Dylan was heading in the right direction and would likely be off Versed in the next twenty-four to thirty-six hours. I immediately felt guilt for allowing myself to relax. I let my guard down. Erica noticed my reaction. I got cranky and depressed. She had a busy day planned with house cleaners coming (a donation from a wonderful a friend), and a counseling appointment for Bella. Bella's world was turned upside down like the rest of us, we can't forget about anyone. I told Erica to forget about bringing me lunch, I could grab a box lunch at the cafeteria. The hospital's idea for COVID restrictions in the cafeteria was prepacked box lunches you can take and leave the hospital to eat.

Erica would not have it though and insisted she would bring my lunch. She brought Bella with her, an idea I was not initially thrilled with. I didn't like any of my kids seeing me upset. Bella was the youngest and I want this to be the least scarring as possible for her. I know she wants to feel involved, but I also want to shield her from as much as I can. It turned out I was wrong for not wanting Bella there. She and Erica not only brought me lunch, but they lifted my spirits, and when I returned to Dylan's room it was the beginning of a few hours of improvement. I got back to the room and Dylan had begun shivering but his fever had dropped to around 100 degrees. He was given some meds to stop the shivering, so I didn't really worry about it. Dylan's body temp was displayed in Celsius on one of the machines, so I had to Google the conversion to get a temperature I understood. He had been around 102, so 100 degrees Fahrenheit was an improvement. I was told the fever could be caused by several things, the worst of which would be an infection. The care team took cultures of Dylan's lungs and did everything to rule infection out. UC Davis is a teaching hospital, so I got to hear the doctor tell his student that you "never want to miss an infection." Some of the infection tests will take up to twenty-four hours to return, so the reduction in Versed was halted while they fight the fever. The other possible causes of a fever could be withdrawal from the Versed and/ or **storming**. What in the seven levels of hell is storming? I very quickly learned that storming in a TBI patient occurs when the brain begins to take back control of the body. The brain can act a little haywire in the beginning. Of course, I am explaining this in the simplest of layman's terms, but this was my understanding at the time and ultimately still is today. What I didn't realize then was how long storming could last. Nobody really understands it, or can control it, they just know that it happens. It is different for every TBI patient. The brain needs to get back in its rhythm and can take a while to begin running correctly. A nurse practitioner who came in felt strongly that Dylan was storming. So that's what I went with. Please God, help Dylan with his storming. The doctors still want to make sure they rule out infection, so basically, they freeze all meds right where they are for twenty-four hours, and we wait.

Today, during one of his breathing tube cleanings, Dylan moved his right arm slightly toward his mouth. There are small signs of improvement here and there. I need to focus on these small signs. Deep down, I always knew there would be setbacks, but I need to minimize my focus on them. I need to focus instead on the positive, keep my faith, and maybe the toughest one for me; accept help. Erica helped me today with bringing Bella to lunch. I need to accept help from those offering it, or I won't make it through this. Another day almost done.

Dylan is down to 7 mg of Versed an hour and hopefully he will be off it completely in another day or two. His cough is stronger. He gagged and bit his breathing tube last night. There is no way I can deal with the big picture. I am keenly aware that I must keep my focus on the present. Deep down, I have always known it would not be a straight shot down the road of improvement. However, I must minimize my focus on anything negative to keep any sanity that I may have left. I need to remain positive and keep my faith. Thank God Erica helped me today. I must do so much of this alone, I need to let people in when they offer their help. This is my new mantra. Tonight will be one week since the accident. I have made it this far. Dylan has made it this far. Our family has made it this far. There will be ups and downs, but we can get through this. I love you, Dylan.

MAY 20, 2020 – EIGHT DAYS SINCE THE ACCIDENT.

Again, this morning was a rough one. There were no text updates from Cindy overnight and when I met with her briefly this morning, I could see she was down. Dylan's fever was not any worse but was not gone. This whole thing is just such a wear on our systems that sometimes you just need to allow yourself to be sad. Sometimes you just **need** to cry, and sometimes you even need to get a little mad. I let it all just get to me a little bit too much and I was depressed and cranky all morning. I felt like the doctors' rounds took forever to get to Dylan, and then I found out that Dr. Z was running the show now. She is the original doctor from the ER who told us this was a life-threatening event for Dylan. It is not that I doubt her abilities as a doctor, but she is less communicative than Dr. M. Now, combine that with my already agitated state, and it didn't make for the best morning. I know how important it is to stay positive. If Dylan can feel any energy in the room, I want it to be positive energy. I want to stay positive, and I will do better at it!!!

I finally received a good update, of course it was an unofficial update from a nurse, which seems to always be where the good news comes from. They have decided to go back to the Versed reduction and to even try to begin reducing some other meds. They have still not been able to identify exactly why Dylan keeps running a fever, but they have ruled out most types of infection, so they feel safe in beginning the medicine reduction again. Dylan had been leaking blood and fluids from his left ear. The main impact of his head hitting the road was directly behind his left ear. The doctors briefed me on some bones poking through something in his ear and this was causing the leaking. This was not a major concern, and honestly at this point appears to be healing, as the leaking has stopped.

They gave Dylan an ultrasound of his brain, which I was able to stay in the room to watch. It took a while and of course it bothered him, so it raised his ICP a little bit. Unfortunately, they believe Dylan may be having some spasms of the blood vessels, so they had to take him for a CT and dye test to check his capillaries. He did ok with the transport and testing, and his ICP went back to his normal range soon after he returned to the room with me. I don't know the results yet, but I am grateful he is back where I can see him. I always need to know that he's okay.

At this point, I made a promise to myself to always recognize and be present in the fact that this is now a journey for me too. I am a fixer. My personality is that I try to fix everything for everyone in my life. I do this to a point that it is a fault of mine and often brings me stress. This is now, by far, the biggest and the worst thing I have ever needed to fix. I constantly stare at his ICPs and check his body temperature readout. I fight with myself over being bothered about how I can fix and control these things. I internalize these feelings of failure when things don't get immediately better, which is hurtful and stressful to me. It wears me down and is utterly exhausting. I must change, right now.

This is now my journey; I need to teach myself to be part of it, not try to control it, or fix it. My job needs to be the positive one, to be supportive and understanding. I need to gather facts from the doctors and nurses and relay the information to literally hundreds of family and friends who are praying and rooting for Dylan. I must learn to keep my faith in God and travel the road as it lays before me. I cannot try to steer everything. I have no idea where this is going. I will just keep praying and walking the path.

A story I once heard was on my mind as I sat isolated in the hospital room with Dylan. A few years ago, I attended a memorial service for a beautiful little angel who graced this world with her presence for only a very short time. Lucy is the daughter of one of Erica's cousins, whom Erica was particularly close with growing up. Lucy was born with severe disabilities and birth defects that shortened her life. Dylan, years before this injury, had been with us when we attended her fourth birthday party. The doctors had said Lucy wasn't expected to make it beyond her first birthday. Despite these disabilities, Lucy seemed able to enjoy her life and showed real happiness in moments. Unfortunately, shortly after that birthday party, Erica and I attended her memorial service. It was obviously a very emotional event. Lucy's parents, Rachelle and Bowen, were incredibly strong at the service and shared something with everyone in attendance. They told a story about how someone had explained to them what their life had become when their daughter was born with her conditions. They said, "Imagine you planned your whole life for a trip to Italy. You learn the language; you love the foods. You study the culture and history and make plans to visit all the wonderful places. You pack your suitcases with everything you need for Italy, and then you get on the plane. When the plane lands, you deboard and you are in **Amsterdam,** not Italy. The language is foreign. The food and climate are different. This is not what you ever planned for or expected, yet here you are. Once you get a moment to reflect, you acknowledge that Amsterdam is beautiful in its own way. Things are different, but you can learn to like it here. It is nothing like you planned for and dreamed of, but that doesn't make it bad. You can learn to like Amsterdam and probably even enjoy it. You just need to modify your expectations and change your perspective." So now we will just adjust to our life with Dylan...in Amsterdam.

Chapter 4

DIRE OUTLOOKS

MAY 22, 2020 — TEN DAYS SINCE THE ACCIDENT.

Yesterday was so busy that journaling never crossed my mind. It started out very frustrating as Dylan's fever was not reducing, and I felt like the doctors were stumped on what to do. Dylan was taken for an MRI overnight but there was a mix up, and he had only gotten a spinal MRI, **not** a brain MRI, which is what he really needed. His spine looks good according to the results, but no one had suspected a spinal injury. I was frustrated about the mix up, and that got me upset. There had been so much improvement the day before. I know I must treat this as a road I have to travel, but what happens when I don't want to do it anymore? I want to be at the end, but of course, I want it to be the ending I want. Dylan could easily have died already, so dealing with this, is better than dealing with the reality of that. I had to leave Dylan's room for a minute and call Erica. She helped me refocus. What would I do without her?! I calmed down, went back in the room and back to walking my road; it is all I can do now. If walking the road means waiting and praying, then that is what I will do. I did a little work on my laptop and kept an eye on Dylan's monitors. Being able to concentrate on work helps take my focus off the machines monitoring Dylan.

The surgeon came in to tell me he reviewed the MRI of Dylan's spine, and everything looked good. He did raise a concern that the area of Dylan's brain, which controls speech, may be impacted by his accident, but admitted that the truth is, he does not really know. I don't really have the time, or energy, for "maybes" right now. I want Dylan to wake up first; then we can worry about deficits. By the afternoon, the care team seemed to have a plan for moving forward. They brought in a machine to cool Dylan's blood and hoped that would help to keep him from shivering. It was incredibly painful to sit in the chair in the corner of the dark hospital room and watch Dylan's body shiver. They could not just heap blankets on him because his temperature was so high. This machine could possibly help cool Dylan's blood and put him near a more normal body temperature. I had to leave the room while they did a little procedure to set it up. I texted everyone about the machine to cool Dylan's blood, and Matthew did some research to see what we were dealing with. Near the end of day one with this new machine, a nurse came in and told me that the charge nurse had agreed to let Matthew and Gabby come in and see their brother for the first time. They could visit him one at a time, but only for a few minutes. The thing we had learned with the COVID rules was that the charge nurse trumped everything. That person was the on-site boss who told us what we could and could not do. We had been bugging the doctors and nurses for days to let them see him, finally we had run into the right charge nurse. I really felt this would be positive for all three of them.

We had to leap at the opportunity to take advantage of the window of a sympathetic charge nurse. That evening, Cindy brought Matthew and Gabby with her to the hospital. I tried one last time to get the charge nurse to let me stay in the room while they visited with him, but she would not budge on that point. I wish it was different, I really wanted to be there to help them. I decided to take what we could get and went down to the lobby to update everyone on Dylan's status and did my best to try to brace them for what they were about to see. Matthew and Gabby took turns going in to see him; Matthew went first. I was super nervous for them to be in there alone. It was very difficult to see Dylan in his puffy comatose state. How would they react? In the end, both Matthew and Gabby came out and were fine. Both said they felt better now that they got to see and touch him. Obviously, Dylan could not speak, but my heart tells me he benefited from the visits also.

Dylan had a good night that night. Maybe it was because of the visit from his brother and sister, maybe it was the blood cooling machine. Most likely, it was a combination of both. Dylan has been at 5 mg/hr of Versed for a few days, so hopefully they get back to slowly reducing it. I feel like he is getting stronger, and if they reduce the Versed, he can finally wake up. I can only pray and keep my eyes on the road.

MAY 23, 2020 – ELEVEN DAYS SINCE THE ACCIDENT.

It was an extremely difficult twenty-four hours. After the surgeon gave me the good update on Dylan's spinal MRI yesterday morning, Dr. Z decided we should have a family update. Due to COVID, they did not want everyone in the hospital, so it was decided that I would be in the conference room with Dr. Z and some other doctors and nurses, while everyone else videoed in on Zoom. Dr. Z gave us **no** indication that anything was wrong and seemed rather upbeat going into the meeting. Then, BOOM! Dr. Z started in with every horrible possibility: **Dylan may never wake from this, he will likely never be independent, won't go to college, may never communicate…**she just kept going. No hope…no "maybes," absolutely nothing positive. This was by far the worst delivery of bad news I had ever been a part of. Because of my career in law enforcement, I have been a part of the delivery of bad news. There is a way to break it more gently, to build up toward the worst parts. This is the opposite of how I believe you do it. Even if it was all true and Dylan never wakes up, this is not how you lay it on a tired and beaten down family. Dr. Z crushed all our hopes in a matter of minutes. It almost felt like that is what she intended to do. I mean, why are we doing this? Is this a pull the plug kind of scenario? She was all negative and provided zero optimism. I know she needed to give us an update and not fill us with false hope, but if she was going to be this negative, she should have clued me in a little before we went live on Zoom with everyone. I could have at least helped to brace my family. The bad news sent Matthew into a tailspin. He seemed inconsolable to me as I watched over the Zoom video feed. I remember Cindy saying something about hope to Dr. Z, but she just killed the idea. Cindy asked if I believed what Dr. Z was saying, but I couldn't answer, if I opened my mouth even a crack, a bellow of sadness would have come out. I just sat there quiet with my mask on, and my eyes full of tears behind my glasses. This made me feel like a failure. I made a note about who was in the room; besides Dr. Z, there was nurse Seph, nurse Katie, and Dr. L. I wondered if they too believed in the bad news. No one had indicated to me at any time that things were this dire. I wondered what their opinions of hope were, but no one else spoke. I couldn't ask because I couldn't speak. I knew then, I would never get over that moment. I would need to speak to a professional counselor about this one. I later spoke with Cindy about this meeting and while it was scarring, we decided to ignore Dr. Z. The nurses, and other doctors who come to Dylan's room, while always being cautious, did give reasons for **hope.** They had seen miracles before. Why can't we get a miracle?

When I got back to the room, they were just finishing up giving Dylan an ultrasound. A short time later Dr. Z, whom I now hated with all my being, came in to tell me the spasms in Dylan's blood vessels have worsened, and Dylan needed a CT scan as soon as possible. They took Dylan away and I went outside and called Erica and cried for the entire hour they had Dylan. I cried, but also came to grips with what Dr. Z had said. She gave all worst-case scenarios, but she could never completely shut the door on this turning out ok. If every story needed a villain, she would be ours. Let's go, Dylan, prove her wrong! Now more than ever, I need to focus on the road, go hour by hour, and let God have all control. Maybe this is the bottom…anything we get from here is better than where we are right now. I must share that message with my family and be the positive energy. No one benefits from sadness and despair. I need to lead my family through this, whatever that means, wherever this goes. That is the reason I am here.

By the time Dylan got back to the room and settled in, the doctors had rotated, and it was Dr. M now. His approach was much better than Dr. Z's; maybe not with what he said, because let's face it, Dylan was in a very bad place, but **how** he said it was much warmer, and made it easier to handle. The spasms in Dylan's brain were worsening, so they need to change up their approach. They are going to increase the Versed again and deepen Dylan's coma. They are going to give him meds to **paralyze** him and hope that helps to stop his shivering. They want to get his temp down to 96 degrees Fahrenheit and wait. Then they will probably leave Dylan like that for two to three days, to give his brain more time to relax and heal. I guess I find some solace in thinking of it like Dylan is not sick, he is not fighting a disease which will likely continue to worsen. He suffered a traumatic injury, but that is over now. Now, his body is fighting to begin healing. It makes me feel like time is more on our side. As I sit here right now, he is healing…slowly, and bit by bit, but he is healing. This is a better way to think of it, or maybe I am just going crazy.

It bothers me how tough this also is on Erica. Yesterday she had to deal with me being very upset, but she couldn't even see me, and we could barely communicate. We were only able to make short calls or text messages because I didn't want to be away from Dylan. It is so hard to share deep emotions that way. After speaking with her when I got home, I realized she is imagining it even worse than it is. She is amazing though, and we talk through everything when I get home, before I fall asleep. I need her strength. I know that together, we will get through this.

MAY 24, 2020 – TWELVE DAYS SINCE THE ACCIDENT.

Dylan has still not improved. Today the concern is mostly with the spasms, as they are getting worse. They are going to do an angioplasty procedure where they go in through his groin and locate the spasms, and either use a balloon or inject medicine right at the point of the spasms to get them to stop. I will admit that I am feeling a little overwhelmed...ok, **a lot overwhelmed.** I feel like Dylan cannot catch a break. I pray for something to give, and for him to improve, even in just one area. It's twelve days since the accident. Today, they are going to try to dilate the blood vessels in his brain and increase the blood flow. I am praying this works. I am praying this is the beginning of some improvements. Today, I sprinkled Dylan with holy water, and I prayed the Rosary. I have not prayed the Rosary since I was a young boy. I recall praying it with my grandmother, at my grandfather's funeral, but that was in the late 1980s. Today, I had to use an app on my phone to walk me through the process. It is a struggle to keep hope, but everyone is helping me. I get texts and emails from friends and family, from all over the world. Even the smallest kind words help. I never knew there was so much power in little messages like that. Those messages help me when I feel weak. Since the last surgery, Dylan has begun to show some improvement, and basically was able to overcome the swelling and ICP problem. I am hoping this procedure can put an end to the spams issue. I know it is serious because the doctors tell me it is, but I would be lying if I said I really understand why the spasms are such a concern right now. With so much stress, it is hard for me to think logically. Of course, a spasming blood vessel inside the brain is not delivering blood to the brain in the proper manner. Lack of blood to the brain is never a good thing. I would love to hear that they can begin reducing the meds again.

When Erica came to have lunch with me, I took the opportunity to ask the nurse if she could come see Dylan for a minute. The persistence paid off and I got a yes. I went and sat in the car and started eating while Erica checked in and made her way to the room. Much like with Matthew and Gabby, I was worried about how she would handle seeing him. Erica came back to the car after a bit with tears streaming down her cheeks. It scared me at first because I thought they were tears of sadness. While there was sadness in the situation, Erica's tears were more of joy because when she walked into Dylan's room and spoke, he turned his head ever so slightly like he heard her voice and was looking for her. There is such hope in moments like this.

MAY 25, 2020 – THIRTEEN DAYS SINCE THE ACCIDENT.

Yesterday morning was another tough one. The report was that the spasms are worsening and that is beginning to make Dylan's pupils sluggish. First thing in the morning Cindy briefed me in the lobby and told me Dylan would be going back in for another procedure around eight a.m. to try to stop the spasms. This procedure was going to be done by a vascular surgeon. They would insert a catheter through Dylan's groin and get into his brain to inject a medicine directly onto the spasms. But eight o'clock came and went and Dylan was not taken anywhere…nine a.m., ten a.m.…nothing. Finally, at 10:30 a.m., I left Dylan's room and went and sat in my truck in the parking garage at UC Davis Hospital. Erica's Auntie Stella and Uncle Jamie had arranged for a Mass to be held in Dylan's honor at their local church, St. Joan of Arc in Victorville, California. The same church where Erica's parents got married. And sadly, the same church where we would attend the memorial service for Uncle Jamie more than a year later when he lost his battle with COVID. The church was hundreds of miles away but it didn't matter since it was COVID. Everyone had to watch the Mass on video anyway. The service was beautiful, and they prayed for Dylan and mentioned him by name several times. It was the Mass of Ascension, so it was full of hope; exactly what I was a little low on at that moment. Erica had driven to the hospital and joined me in my truck to watch the service on my iPad. She also brought me lunch, which she did every single day…not just for the food, but for the brief break in my twelve-hour vigils.

I got back to Dylan's room around 12:30, and the nurse told me there was STILL no response from the surgeon about Dylan's procedure. I was wondering if I should start making some demands and getting some answers. If Dylan needs this now, then I want it done now! I let the nurse know I was not happy, and he contacted Dr. Z and the vascular surgeon resident, who was ironically named Dylan. The resident came to the room and told me the surgery was not considered an emergency, and it would be done in the next day or two. Not an emergency? It sure seemed like the neurological team felt like it was an emergency. I had just typed out a long text to inform everyone about the delay in the procedure, when the resident came back in the room and told me that Dr. Z had personally contacted the vascular surgeon, and he was on his way to the hospital. I never mean to imply that Dr. Z didn't care about Dylan. It was her poor delivery of the dire unknown outcome which we all had hated.

They immediately started prepping Dylan and took him away. By 1:30, I was in my truck taking a nap. I usually cannot nap, but I fell asleep and slept until 3:15. Let's be honest, I passed out from exhaustion. Then, I walked to the local Starbucks for a nitro coffee. It was the same Starbucks we walked to during Dylan's second surgery. They had tables in front of the door so no one could enter. The staff took your order and then delivered your drink to the table so you could walk away without ever entering—more COVID coldness. I was on the phone with Erica while walking back to the hospital, when my phone beeped that I had a voicemail; Dylan was back in his room. I got back to him as quickly as possible. When I walked in, I thought he looked a little puffy, but otherwise, he seemed to be resting peacefully.

The nurse practitioner began giving me an update but as he was talking to me, Dr. Z walked in. She had a mask on, but I believe under it, she was smiling. She said the procedure went "better than expected." Apparently, the surgeon said it was not as bad as they had feared when he got into Dylan's brain. She said the procedure gives them a better look at the brain than an MRI or a CT scan. She also said they were able to stop the spasms. The original plan was to leave the catheter in place in his brain, but based on what they saw, they decided to remove it at the end of the procedure. They were confident they would not need to go back in, at least not for the next twenty-four to forty-eight hours. Now, Dylan just needed to rest.

MAY 26, 2020 – FOURTEEN DAYS SINCE THE ACCIDENT.

Come on, Dylan!!!! We are all so filled with worry. We have all accepted that we don't know what the future holds. We know life has forever changed from where we all thought we were heading; you were going off to play college football and us getting one step closer to an empty nest. Now we just want you alive, we want you with us. We want you out of this coma, so we can have some interaction with you.

Yesterday was mostly boring. They tried to reduce the paralytic, but Dylan immediately began shivering again. They tried to control the shivering with Demerol, but that only worked for about fifteen minutes. So now he is back on the paralytic, back to resting, and we will try again tomorrow.

MAY 27, 2020 – FIFTEEN DAYS SINCE THE ACCIDENT.

The shivers again! I hate these things, and I cannot wait until we beat them. This morning, they tried stopping the paralytic again, and immediately the shivers came back. They are trying a drug combination to try to control them, Demerol or Dilaudid, and some other medicine for pain. I know Dylan won't remember the pain, but it hurts me to see him shiver. Is it because of the pain? Is it the fever? No one can tell me for sure. I just want them to go away. I feel like these shivers are what is holding us back now. This also feels like it is 100 percent related to one of the most terrifying nightmares I had as a child. The nightmare doesn't sound scary, but the feeling I got from it terrified me my entire life, and now it is here. It's the shivering! My nightmare consisted of me in a giant football stadium. The stadium was empty, and it was surrounded on the outside by giant rock cliffs, like something you would see in Hawaii. I was at the very top of the stadium and I was gliding down the walkway, toward the field. There were steps, but I wasn't walking, I was gliding over the steps. If I was gliding smoothly, everything was peaceful, but every now and then, the gliding shook. I shivered and I would get terrified. I was trying anything to keep the gliding smooth but there really was no way. Every now and then, a terrifying shiver came along and shot a jolt of fear through me. I was probably around ten years old when I had that nightmare, and I can still relate to the terror I felt. No boogey man, no zombies. Just the feeling of these shivers, and now here they are in my real life…in the most terrifying way possible, affecting my child.

All I want right now is for Dylan to rest peacefully and begin his road to recovery, but every now and then, he shivers. I would try anything to control them, and the doctors are trying everything to control them, but no matter what we do, eventually he returns to shivering. This really is my nightmare playing out in real life. Was the nightmare from forty years ago really a premonition that I would one day be going through this in real life? That nightmare stopped when I eventually woke up. When will Dylan wake up?

Trying to focus on the positive...I would say they have slowed the shivers down. They don't seem to come as often, as I watch from my cold, dark chair in the corner. I believe the shivering may be connected to the pain meds and I hope they eventually find the right combination to help him. Dylan may be addicted to Oxycontin before this is all over, but I will take my chances beating that, to get him through this. I just want to take him fishing!

Dylan loved fishing even more than most kids. He taught Ty to fish, and the two of them would walk to local ponds on a regular basis and see what was biting. Dylan also had a knack for fishing. It was very rare that anyone would catch more fish than he did. I took Matthew and Dylan camping and fishing for Dylan's twelfth birthday. The three of us lined up chairs evenly spaced apart on the shore of lake and started fishing for trout. Dylan was in the middle. A few hours later, Dylan had six keeper-sized trout on the stringer and Matthew and I had not caught a single fish between us. As we were leaving, a lady asked is we minded if she moved to Dylan's spot to try to catch her first fish of the day. We didn't mind but we highly doubted she would have Dylan's luck.

MAY 29, 2020 – SEVENTEEN DAYS SINCE THE ACCIDENT.

My birthday, not the most desirable way to spend one, but I was not going to miss a day in the hospital. I certainly had no desire to celebrate anything. Yesterday started out like the day before, with the shivers being mostly uncontrolled. The doctors decided to begin lowering the Versed, and now Dylan shivered whenever he was stimulated. I just wanted to keep everyone from touching him. I was a little depressed since there really had not been much improvement of any kind the past few days. Erica brought me lunch and I met her at a nearby park to eat. That always lifts my spirits a little. She always fights so hard to brighten my day. We had begun feeding a few squirrels with our leftovers, and now they seemed to join us for lunch most days. After lunch, I was back in Dylan's room and Dr. K came in to check on Dylan. I believe Dr. K was a resident. Dr. K was young and tall and kind of sounded like he had a New York accent. We spoke about Dylan's shivering, and he was able to observe it firsthand. Dr. K ordered the nurse to put socks on Dylan's hands and feet. The nurse questioned the order, saying, "I don't think that is the issue," but Dr. K responded with, "When I shiver with fever, I want socks, gloves, and a blanket. So, let's try it." The nurse put socks on Dylan's hands and feet and got him an extra blanket, and almost immediately, the shivering improved. It was effective if you ask me. It worked well for the next hour or so, until they came in to do an echocardiogram. Dylan did not respond well to being stimulated and the shivers naturally came back.

The reason for the echocardiogram was they were concerned with how bloated Dylan had become. They wanted to lower Dylan's hydration but the better hydrated you are, the more elasticity the blood vessels have. Dylan needed elasticity in his blood vessels while he was having those spasms. Since the spasms had improved, they wanted to address the bloating now. Dr. S did the echocardiogram and because this was a teaching hospital, he had several students in the room. He commented how remarkably healthy Dylan's heart was and added: "As you would expect from a scholarship athlete."

Dylan did shiver all through the echocardiogram, but otherwise did well. In the middle of the procedure, Dr. S noticed the socks on Dylan's hands and feet and asked, "Who did this?" Dr. K sort of shyly raised his hand. Dr. S asked the nurse if Dylan's shivering had improved with the socks on, and she said she had been very busy and had not noticed a difference. I typically just sat quietly in the corner of the room, but I decided to speak up. I called out that I felt that his shivering had lessened. Dr. S was very personable and friendly, and sought more of my input on Dylan. He pointed out to his students that no one sees Dylan more than the parents in the room twenty-four hours a day, so getting feedback from me, he said, was very important. He was the first doctor to really make me feel like I was serving a purpose. Nurses had done it before, but this was new. Dr. S also made sure to thank, and congratulate, Dr. K for his wonderful idea. THIS is the kind of positive energy I want around Dylan. I want to feel like I am being helpful, and I want Dylan to be surrounded by people looking for the positives. Dr. S is tall, fit, and charismatic. You know every time he walks in the room, and he just emits positive energy. This energy not only helped me to feel better, but Dylan's shivers also decreased, so finally there is something to consider as improvement.

Speaking of positive attitudes, Cindy and I have begun discussing having Dr. Z removed from Dylan's care team. One nurse confided in Cindy that Dr. Z was not her favorite doctor, and another nurse informed her that we always have the right to remove someone from Dylan's care team. I spoke with my mom and my sister about this, and also with Erica, Matthew, and Gabby. We all decided that the next day, I would ask to meet with a hospital administrator to ask for Dr. Z to be removed from Dylan's care team. That night, as I was getting ready for bed, Cindy texted me to let me know that Dr. Z was there putting a new central line in Dylan. I wasn't comfortable with it, but there was not much I could do now. Cindy eventually said the procedure went very well and she ended up speaking with Dr. Z about Dylan's chances of recovery. Dr. Z had been so negative in that family meeting that we were all scarred from it and wanted her gone. However, Cindy now felt Dr. Z had an attitude filled with a little more hope this time they spoke.

The next morning, Dr. S came into Dylan's room, and we spoke for almost thirty minutes about the decision to give Dylan the central line. He explained how the decision was made, and why. Dr. S assured me that Dylan's current group of doctors are a **team,** and that **everyone** has input on the care decisions that occur. I felt better about Dr. Z now, knowing how the decisions were being made. I never thought Dr. Z did anything wrong medically, it was just the conflicts in personality and bedside manner. I would not have hesitated to question things, if I thought her medical decisions were as bad as her delivery. I spoke with everyone again, and we decided to hold off on making any changes to Dylan's care team. Not liking someone's delivery is different than not believing in their abilities. We are all under a great deal of stress. We will just ask that any future family updates should come from a different doctor.

Now I want to be sure I write about the power of prayer. I have prayed all my life, but never anything like this. I have never in my life asked for prayers before, and now I find myself asking everyone I speak with. I hear about prayer groups from all over the United States, and even the world, praying for Dylan. I have blessed Dylan's room with holy water and relearned how to pray the Rosary. Our friends Taunya and Gene text us beautiful prayers every day, often multiple times a day, from both themselves and people in their prayer group. I believe in my heart and soul that the prayers are helping Dylan. I also know for sure they are helping me. This is something I can do…something I can focus on. It helps to calm me down and to give me strength. I don't think I could sit at Dylan's side every day, for twelve hours a day, without the strength of those prayers.

MAY 30, 2020 – EIGHTEEN DAYS SINCE THE ACCIDENT.

Dylan seems to finally be making some progress. He is down to 6 mg per hour on the Versed, and some other drugs have also been lowered. He appears to be resting more peacefully. The doctors had to stop using the blood cooling machine, I am not sure why. This allowed his fever to climb back to 101 and again made it a point of concern. Dylan is scheduled for another CT scan tonight and I am nervous and anxious for what they will find. I have these lingering effects of Dr. Z filling my head with dreadful thoughts of what Dylan's life may look like after this. The unknown is the hardest part. It is my constant fight to stay positive and remind myself that this is at least a six-month journey. I tell myself that I will have won the lottery if we just get him back to a functioning young man, who can laugh, and who I can take fishing. Of course, I hope for the best, but Dr. Z made that hard. I will always hold some ill will toward her for that. I just need to trust in God and keep praying to one day hear his laugh again.

Chapter 5

A SURPRISE VISITOR

What a rollercoaster ride this is! Leaving here last night, I was concerned because the Versed level was getting lower, but we were not seeing any movement. The first time they lowered the Versed I felt like there was a little more movement from him. My worries only increased the next morning when I woke up and there were no text updates from Cindy. I always take her silence as a bad sign. I woke up at two a.m. and couldn't fall back to sleep. I just laid there worrying that he may not come out of this. When I got to the hospital and met with Cindy, she seemed extra depressed. I mentioned not seeing any movement, and she agreed with me. I mostly just took one anxiety pill at night so I could sleep, but this day I needed to take half of a pill just to be able to stop crying. I was also leery of the giant dark cloud on the horizon, the report from Dylan's overnight CT scan. Was it just going to be more forecasting of doom from Dr. Z?

The morning started off slow. I sat in the chair in the corner of the room and fought off tears; a mostly losing battle. Late that morning, I noticed a single cough from Dylan, all on his own. Soon after, the nurse was putting some drops in Dylan's eyes and Dylan tried to turn away, yet another good sign. Next, the surgeons came in and commented that Dylan was having some increased reactions to light in his pupils. They also said Dylan was not draining as much fluid from his brain, and that they were able to raise the fluid drain from ten to fifteen. They told me that when the drain goes to twenty, it can come out. I was not exactly sure what all this meant, but it all sounded positive. They said he is still critical but is now heading in the right direction.

Soon after the surgeons left, Dr. S came in the room, and I immediately told him about Dylan's eyes. He seemed surprised. He pinched Dylan hard on the chest and Dylan raised both arms. Finally, a documentable encouraging sign. There is hope! Dr. S explained that the Versed can be stored in fatty tissue and may take twenty-four hours to fully leave Dylan's system once it is stopped. Dylan was on Versed for close to three weeks with levels as high as 40 mg per hour. When Dr. S left, I prayed the Rosary and sprinkled Dylan with holy water. Over the next few hours, there were more good signs. Dylan pulled away when the breathing tube was cleaned, I saw his nose wiggle, and he even yawned. He was not yet conscious, but he was getting there.

JUNE 1, 2020 – TWENTY DAYS SINCE THE ACCIDENT.

Today, there is more of this rollercoaster! When Cindy relieved me, she went to say hello to Dylan and grabbed his hand. Dylan not only opened his eyes for her, but he pulled her hand toward his chest. Great news except the downside to that though, was that his heart raced to 171 beats per minute. They immediately gave him some drugs to calm him down. Maybe he is starting to wake up and is getting scared. Cindy spent the rest of the night staying quiet and letting him rest. This morning, I was finally given the results of the CT scan from the other night, and it was some decent news. It looks like the spasms have stopped. Unfortunately, on this rollercoaster there is never only good news. They told me that since he is not yet awake, he is going to need a tracheotomy. They had warned us this day may come, but of course we had hoped to avoid it. I am not sure why I see it as such a bad thing, maybe because it just feels more permanent to me. Will he ever get it removed down the road? Just last night, I was bragging about how he had not needed to have one. I mean, you can just never relax on this road; something always lurks around the bend.

When the care team came in for the morning rounds, they noticed that Dylan had bit off a piece of his breathing tube; the small balloon which holds it in place. He would either need to have a new breathing tube inserted, or have the trach put in today. Dr. S and the nurse practitioner explained the choices and the procedure to me in extensive detail. Mostly, because I was questioning everything. They emphasized that Dylan is breathing on his own, and that he often breathes over the machine itself. His lungs are very strong. They fully see this trach as just a temporary thing. When Dylan wakes up more and begins rehabilitating, he will have the trach removed and the hole in his skin will heal itself over time. The trach was clearly the better option over a new breathing tube, which has higher risks and chances of possible side effects. I am clinging to the word **"temporary."** No one made any promises, but they at least gave room for hope! They also said, **"When he gets to rehab,"** and to me…that's more positive thoughts.

Life changed for a lot of people on the night of May 12, 2020, but that doesn't now necessarily mean it will be a bad life. Erica is helping me stay positive, and stresses to be sure we enjoy each victory. Dylan is alive. There had been some progress and he **is** slowly improving. No one can tell how much he will improve, or how far he can go. Not even the experts. Unfortunately, there are plenty of examples of people who lost their loved ones and didn't get a chance to have any hope to have them back. I heard of a five-year-old boy who drowned last weekend. Being able to fight this with Dylan is a blessing; there is hope. We will enjoy every little improvement and keep walking the road.

JUNE 2, 2020 – TWENTY-ONE DAYS SINCE THE ACCIDENT.

When I got home last night, I got a great surprise! My brother Todd was there. He had flown in from Pennsylvania. Erica had surprised me and arranged for him to come help. As soon as I saw him, I hugged him and became overwhelmed with tears and emotion. Eventually, I got my wits about me. It felt great to have someone else there, even if he could do very little. Without my knowing, Erica had arranged with Cindy to switch shifts, so Cindy was going to cover the next twenty-four straight hours with Dylan, and then I would be on the night shift. I got to sleep in a little bit the next morning and then wake up and spend some more time visiting with my brother. We did some much-needed little chores around the house and then spent some time relaxing in the pool. It seemed like just a few minutes before it was time for my first night shift, but the relief was great. It was a small slice of normal, and I'm grateful.

I guess a part of me has always believed a little bit in seeing signs. I recall a story my mom told me about a cardinal that appeared outside the bedroom window of my grandmother's bedroom, as she rested on home hospice the last few days of her life. To my mom, that cardinal was my grandfather comforting her. As we relaxed in the pool with my brother, we noticed a blue bird hanging around. The blue bird stayed with us all day long, I had never noticed it hanging around before. My mom then told us the blue bird is a sign of hope. I will take it; I will believe in that hope.

Dylan has made some medical progress. His meds and equipment have been reduced. There seemed like much more space in his room because there is significantly less equipment. He was still running a bit of a fever and was on a large amount of pain killers, but the fear of him dying at any moment had been greatly reduced. Now I can begin to think just a little bit about his recovery. Dylan has a very long, long way to go. I know it will be slow, but I am hopeful. Whenever I get too down, I just need to look back at this journal to read about how BAD things were—the endless times I spent praying that he just makes it through the night. I have hope that we can make a happy life for him, in whatever form that may be.

JUNE 3, 2020 – TWENTY-TWO DAYS SINCE THE ACCIDENT.

I don't even think I can journal anymore. I just don't have the energy to write. The word from the doctors today is that Dylan is not progressing as he should. This is not a total shock, as we can see he is not moving. I can only keep praying and hoping that Dylan is moving at his own slow pace. He always did march to the beat of his own drum; I would expect him to do things at his own rate. The staff told me he may be transported to a Kaiser Permanente Hospital soon. Since Kaiser is my insurance, they will move him to one of their hospitals as soon as he is stable enough to go. The doctors said it could be as soon as tomorrow. Dylan can squeeze my hand as I speak to him, so I am in no way ready to give up yet. I am tired and I am broken. These are the hardest words I have ever written in my life...**please Jesus, don't let him suffer. I want him happy and safe, at your side...or mine.** If you must take him away, then let it be now. We have already all suffered so much through this. We cannot possibly have come this far...only to come this far.

JUNE 5, 2020 – TWENTY-FOUR DAYS SINCE THE ACCIDENT.

I skipped a day of journaling. This night shift is a different animal and can go by quick. I did some work on my laptop and then fell asleep before I could journal. "Sleep" may be the wrong term, but I put on my headphones and tried to rest in my cold, dark corner. I close my eyes and wait to detect movement in the room to know when the nurse is there. I wish I would have journaled though because it was a good day. The overwhelming feeling from the day before had worked its way through all of us. Yesterday was better. Dylan made some small improvements, and I was able to accept things as they are. Better to be where we are today, than where we were last week; better to be where we are today, than yesterday. Today at 6:30 a.m., my high school friend, Bill Fetterolf, texted me "I love you." That caused a burst of emotion in me. Bill lost his teenaged son, Chandler, to suicide and one year ago today was the funeral. It breaks my heart to hear how deeply it still affects Bill. But of course, it does…I can't imagine that it ever won't. I can relate now more than ever, with what he must have gone through, and is still going through. I am sure there is no real end to it, and that is likely what my future holds. No matter what the outcome, life has changed. I wish I had been a better friend for Bill when it first happened. I feel very guilty for that. Now I see the value of what true friendship like that means. I was always more of a "give them space" kind of person, but when Dylan's accident hit, it turns out that I needed the **help** of family and friends, not **space.** Even if there is nothing anyone can do, nice words help in some small way. It gives me some strength to have someone like Bill as a friend. Someone who has gone through something similar and has such an understanding. I don't feel like I must explain my feelings to him because he knows. With that comes some weird kind of guilt that Dylan is still here. Dylan can squeeze my hand, and Bill and others who have lost children will never get that. Does anyone ever sit in my seat and call themselves lucky?

My brother left today, and it made for a slower day. I can't stress enough how nice it was to have him here and how much I needed it. COVID has really made this journey harder and forced me and Cindy to do more by ourselves. Family and friends can help us at home, but if not for COVID, they could help so much more. But I won't allow myself to dwell on this. It is just another thing I cannot change. My brother's visit lifted my spirits, and I will do my best to keep them there. The nurses caring for Dylan tonight were positive thinkers, so that also helps. It means so much when they tell me stories of other patients who have been through these rooms and halls and have gotten better.

JUNE 6, 2020 – TWENTY-FIVE DAYS SINCE THE ACCIDENT.

Last night was not a good night. I fell asleep and woke up at three a.m. with Dylan's ventilator sounding an alarm. Dylan stormed relentlessly for the next several hours. His heart rate would go up to 177 bpm at times and his fever spiked. For some reason, this kept setting off his ventilator alarm. I tried to calm him with touch and words, but nothing worked. The nurses paged the on-call doctors, and they prescribed pain killers and Versed for him. The Versed helped a little, but when I left at six a.m., he was still not resting comfortably. Cindy took over for the day and around 11:30 a.m. she noticed his belly seemed hard. She pointed it out to the nurse, and an ultrasound revealed Dylan's bladder was extremely full. They changed Dylan's catheter and once he was able to relieve his bladder, he became much more restful.

When I saw him again the next night, I could tell he was somewhat calm again, and he looked less bloated. When I got to his room and began speaking with the nurse, I noticed Dylan raised his left hand just a little. I believe he recognized my voice and reached for me. That is the greatest feeling in the world right now. What a surge of emotions. One minute, we are screaming downhill, and the next, there are new highs. How do you survive this? Dylan still does not follow commands, but I believe it will come.

The support from family and friends remains incredible. It is crazy how many people seem to be worried about me, as much as they are about Dylan. It never really occurred to me to feel sorry for myself, or complain about the accident, or what I was having to go through. I feel like any parent would do what I am doing. We all pray we never have to do something like this, but my number came up and it was my unfortunate turn. Maybe it is easier for me in some way because I am going through it, and I don't really have time to reflect. Those watching and being told they can't help because of COVID can do only that… **watch.** I have spent long hours praying Dylan would live, and now that that is much more likely, I can begin to focus on what life might eventually be like. I am the type of person to keep my expectations low. Of course, a full recovery would be awesome, but in my heart, I know it is very unlikely there won't be at least a little deficit. If Dylan can experience joy and happiness again, then I know it is something I can live with. If he can express those things, then I would be truly blessed. Right now, I pray and thank God for every little step. Today's step is a rather large one. Dylan is officially off the actual ventilator, and just on some moisturizing vent, which increases the amount of oxygen in the air he breathes. The doctor said we would try it for one hour, and then go back on the ventilator; but six hours passed, and Dylan was still going strong. Go Dylan! This is a big step, and it makes me happy. I just want to soak in that happiness for a few minutes and not think about anything else.

JUNE 7, 2020 – TWENTY-SIX DAYS SINCE THE ACCIDENT.

I met with Dr. M today, and to sum it up, Dylan's brain is damaged in several places. Dr. M stated he would expect Dylan to have disabilities for the rest of his life. The truth of it though, he has no way to know what the extent of those disabilities may be. The doctors don't know Dylan from before the accident, so they don't know how physically strong he was. Dylan is also just about to turn eighteen; the research for brain injuries shows the young heal better, and quicker, than people who are older. What everyone can agree on though, is that Dylan is on a very long journey, not days or months, but years. We are all on that journey with him. We are very lucky to have him alive, and we need to keep focused on the positive. We need to be strong as a family; one big, weird, blended family. Matthew, Gabby, Tyler, Annabella, Zach, and Josh need to be able to grow up as happy young people seeking out their dreams and enjoying life.

Dylan has already come a long way. I have met so many wonderful doctors, nurses, and technicians, and I would be doing them a great disfavor if I only wrote about Dr. Z, or my bad experiences. I have watched them all work together, to **literally** save this boy's life.

JUNE 9, 2020 – TWENTY-EIGHT DAYS SINCE THE ACCIDENT.

Dates and days of the week blur together anymore. I don't sleep right, or eat right, or ever think of anything else. But with that said, we are on the cusp of change on this journey. For the first time, the surgeons have ruled that Dylan **"localized"** to stimulus. This is a big and wonderful step, because it confirms for me that he is progressing, and that's really all I can ask for at this point. It is extremely hard to stay positive if I don't see some progress. I want to stay strong, but I need progress. I fight to keep my faith, and I keep praying and trusting in God.

Today is likely the day Dylan will be transferred to another Kaiser facility. We knew this day would arrive, and like most things along this road, fear of the unknown is the worst fear. We are at UC Davis Hospital in Sacramento, which is a highly respected and extremely well-renowned facility. Kaiser has several hospitals around the area, and I liked them as my insurance, because it was always easy to get an appointment for the little things—cold symptoms, sprained ankles, etc. But this is a whole new ball game. We are comfortable (as much as we can possibly be) at UC Davis. Dylan is improving here…but now we face the unknown. If the world was fair and everyone just truly wanted Dylan to have the best treatment, I believe he would be staying right here. This is an insurance move, not a move to benefit Dylan's recovery as far as I'm concerned. I know this is how health insurance works, but that doesn't mean I have to agree with it. No one can even tell me what facility Dylan is going to. In my heart, I believe Dylan can handle this, but should he have to? Compared to when he first got here, the nurses now must barely pay attention to Dylan. At one point in time, he had two nurses assigned JUST to him, and now, he is just another patient, part of a rotation of patients. I want to get Dylan to a rehab and see what they can do for him. I have no doubt there will be hoops to jump through for the insurance company, but we will get through them. I feel like there is quite a team with great support behind Dylan, and I will use every single resource I can to get Dylan what he needs. I will keep my faith in God and keep hope at the front of my mind. I will do my best to smash my doubts as they arise and to stay positive.

Chapter 6

A CHANGE OF SCENERY

JUNE 10, 2020 – TWENTY-NINE DAYS SINCE THE ACCIDENT.

Dylan was transferred yesterday by an ambulance service. Today is my first day in the Kaiser-Morse Hospital in Sacramento. Of course, a new hospital means new COVID rules. There will be new security guards to fight our way through, and new administrative staff to convince that their COVID rules are nonsensical. How to enter the hospital, visiting hours, and who can visit will all have to be established again. It is another exhausting part of this journey, and one I really don't care to deal with.

I believe the physical toll has finally caught up with me. I have a constant burning in my stomach. It is a constant burning pain, and I don't ever feel any relief. I set up a telephone appointment with my physician and snuck out of Dylan's room take the call. The doctor's advice was to use over-the-counter heartburn meds and call back if it is not better in a few days. I have had heartburn before and this is not what this feels like, but I had no energy to disagree. I hope it gets better soon.

Matthew started a GoFundMe page for Dylan last night, and within the first twenty-four hours it brought in $25,000!! It brings me to tears to see the generosity, such a beautiful outpouring of love for my dear child. There were large donations from family and friends. There were small donations of five dollars, some of which were from children. It causes me to rediscover the humanity in this world. The quarterback Dylan sacked to save the game against the rival football school even donated. The love is real, and it is beautiful. The scary side of this is that we really need that money for Dylan.

This afternoon, I again find myself fighting my demons of doubt. I prayed the Rosary and blessed Dylan and his new room with holy water. I have been told that he needs to progress to the point of following some simple commands, or they won't take him at a rehab facility. He is in ICU at the new hospital, but we hope he gets moved to a regular room soon.

I have learned about something called the **Ranchos Los Amigo's Levels of Cognitive Functioning.** There are eight stages on the scale and making it to stage two on the scale was what the surgeons were excited about. When Dylan had that localized movement after the doctor pinched his chest, it gave them the confirmation they needed. Stage three is the **localized response** stage, and the important part of that is the ability to follow simple commands. We need Dylan at this stage before they will authorize him to go to a rehab facility. A doctor did have the **"what ifs"** talk with me today about what we may have to do if Dylan doesn't progress, and there is just no good answer for that. Every option is bad. There is something called sub-acute care, which I believe is basically like a nursing home. Dylan simply **must** progress. I guess I could handle a temporary care place, but not if he is totally unresponsive; that may be too much for me. I don't know what I would do. But for now, I need to think positive thoughts and help Dylan make as much progress as possible. Dear Lord, let's please make that stage three level of response happen, please.

JUNE 12, 2020 – THIRTY-ONE DAYS SINCE THE ACCIDENT.

Time is just grinding along. Dylan is not progressing fast enough for me, but at least Dylan has not had any major setbacks. I guess that is progress in some way. Internally, I believe he is getting stronger, but I have trouble keeping the grim predictions from Dr. Z out of my head. I fight those thoughts, but a long shift alone in a quiet room gives the mind a lot of time to wander into bad neighborhoods. I know that only God knows where this is going. The doctors have all done their jobs to this point, now we need to wait and see. Negative thoughts at this point do not do anyone any good. Recently I also had to do something else I had never done—contact a therapist. I am lucky enough to have an expanded mental health care coverage at my work. I have previously received emails reminding me that we have the coverage, but I never expected to use it. The emails always say we have therapists available with one simple call. I made that call. I had my first therapy session yesterday, but of course this is COVID, so I could not be seen in person. It was a video call, which I took in the parking lot of a park near the hospital. I think being in person would have been better, but at least it was something. Erica took the call with me, and we cried as we relayed our horrible living nightmare to the therapist. The therapist recommended that when I felt myself becoming stressed about the future, I should try to bring up a memory from the recent past: the ICPs, the surgeries, the shivering. I will focus on the thoughts like that of a week ago when Dylan was not even stable. He was still on the ventilator at UC Davis Hospital. I want him to respond to simple commands so badly that I forget how far he has come. The therapist also repeatedly said, "At least he is here," and that is a truth I need to **never** forget. Dylan being here is all I, along with a lot of friends, family, and strangers, was praying for two or three weeks ago. Let's keep this to one step at a time. I will keep working to develop Dylan's ability to follow simple commands every minute that he is awake.

Anytime Dylan is alert, I work with him to do things on command. I know Cindy does similar things when she is with him. His left thumb seems to be where the movement is beginning to come back. I move his thumb for him and then try to get him to move it on his own. I try to tell him jokes to get a laugh or give him kisses to see if he will move his lips. Dylan holds the tennis ball that nurse Toby put in his hand when he was first at UC Davis Hospital. Most of the time, Dylan holds onto it with his left hand. When he is awake, I sometimes take it from him and try to make him reach to get it back. He gets constant attention from us whenever he is awake. This family will get Dylan through this.

JUNE 13, 2020 – THIRTY-TWO DAYS SINCE THE ACCIDENT.

Today my schedule changed a little. We finally got permission from Kaiser administration to have Matthew and Gabby take some shifts sitting by Dylan's side. When Dylan first moved to Kaiser-Morse, they originally told us we would have to abide by their strict adult visiting hours. We immediately argued that he is a minor, so we should get twenty-four-hour access. We won that argument. We have learned with COVID that the rules are not necessarily finite; if one person says no, just find their boss. Just like Dylan is doing, we keep fighting. I hope Matthew and Gabby are strong enough for this. It is tough, and I don't want my other children to suffer any more than they already have. Like a lot of things along this journey, I underestimated their strength also. We all just really want Dylan to progress and reach that stage three, but there is really nothing we can do but sit and wait. Sitting by his side is great because you get to see him, it is also quite painful for the exact same reason. Physically, Dylan has a misshapen head with indents on both sides where his skull plates have been removed, it is tough to see the first few times. We all know this must be done. Dylan always needs someone in his room, we all agree on that. Now Cindy and I can finally have a little help. Dylan will advance at his own pace, and I am trying to be at peace with that. All I can do, all each of us can do, is our own little part. Patience is tough for me; I desperately want to do more.

Today we also learned that Dylan is positively influenced by music. Unlike weeks ago, when any stimulation sent him into a downward spiral, he seems to wake up and become more alert when we play music. We now have a playlist of about twenty songs that his friends and siblings put together. Some of the songs have some more aggressive lyrics than I might like, so I pause or skip them if someone comes in. I hope playing the music is having the effect of stimulating Dylan's brain to grow and remap. That is certainly what we all hope. This road is terrifying and frustrating, but no one really knows where it leads. I guarantee you that as I read my journal back, I will gladly take sitting here listening to questionable lyrics over his machines beeping at me. Thank you, Jesus, for getting us this far.

JUNE 14, 2020 – THIRTY-THREE DAYS SINCE THE ACCIDENT.

There is new hope today. I admit I was fighting the depression when I came into the hospital this morning, but Dylan was moved out of ICU overnight and is now in a regular room. The move was expected, but like with so many things on this journey, I worry that they may be giving up on Dylan a little. Then again, there is always something to worry about. The doctors seem concerned with the lack of progress, and don't seem to get as excited about the little things, like music stimulation. I know that it is probably not true, and they have not done anything blatant along those lines. I'm sure it's just my anxious, tired brain. The good news is that the regular room is much quieter than the ICU room. Dylan is in a private room and thank God for that. It feels large for a hospital room, and it is nice and secluded. I sat in yet another uncomfortable hospital chair and prayed the Rosary.

Sometimes we need to just let Dylan rest. Around nine a.m., I decided to try to wake Dylan up with some music. I played his playlist, and as usual it stirred him awake a little. I sat by his bedside and asked him to raise his thumb, and he did it! It was his left thumb, and to me, it had noticeably moved. I kept speaking with him and asking him to repeat the movement, and I then saw both hands twitch and move at different times. This is absolute progress and really raises my hopes that Dylan's brain can heal. I know it is small, tiny movements and they are certainly not consistent enough, but this is the most movement I have seen from Dylan since the accident, and damn it…I am celebrating it.

JUNE 17, 2020 – THIRTY-SIX DAYS SINCE THE ACCIDENT.

Another good day yesterday. During the afternoon the nurses got Dylan into something called the cardiac chair. I have no idea where that name originates from, but it has nothing to do with the heart as far as I can see. The staff can slide Dylan onto the chair when it is reclined and then they can move him to a true sitting position. His body is strapped in, so he doesn't slide out. Dylan responded well to not being in a bed for the first time in over a month. While in the chair, he reached for his trach, reached for his catheter, and pulled the little sensor off his right finger using his left hand. I got some video of him moving, and I was able to share it in the text threads. This video is priceless. Video has now become a very important part of this. We all record every little victory we can get and share them via group text threads. Later that night, we got a text from Cindy saying she was able to get him to stick out his tongue on command. Unfortunately, she was not able to get him to repeat it for a video. I can't wait to try to get him to do it for me. It was around this time that I began playing thumb wars with Dylan when he was awake. "One, two, three, four, I declare a thumb war." When he was conscious, Dylan would slowly move his thumb around to avoid me and understood that if he got on top of my thumb, he needed to squeeze me down. Some days he can do it and some days he cannot.

We had a tough day at home yesterday. Apparently, Erica had drama with Ty and Bella and had to get her parents, Nani and Papi, involved. I feel bad that I can't help. There is no way I can do anything from the hospital. Erica purposefully didn't tell me about it until I got home. It is hard for me to get too worked up about teenage drama at this point. I have raised teenagers through normal times, and it can certainly be trying, but I know it will pass. This is laborious for all of us. The truth is, I am highly preoccupied with everything going on with Dylan, but I love all my kids, and I must rely so heavily on Erica to hold down the home front. I know it's not easy. Even with the extra struggles, I am very happy with the blessings we have received so far with Dylan, and I pray he can continue down this path. I will do everything in my power to get Dylan the best care he can get, no matter what!

It was also around this time that a good friend of mine, Mike Chavez, texted me while I was at the hospital and offered to do anything he could to help. The old me would have said, "Thank you, but I am fine." But that guy is gone. I immediately knew of a way he could help. A few hours later, Mike showed up at my house with an arm full of roses. Erica loves flowers; they are part of her love language. She was helping me and maintaining everything domestic, while I spent almost every waking moment in the hospital. I really wanted to bring her some joy, and from what I heard, Mike got a tearful hug for the gesture.

JUNE 19, 2020 – THIRTY-EIGHT DAYS SINCE THE ACCIDENT.

We keep taking steps down our road, but sometimes they are miniscule. Dylan is moving his hands with more regularity, and even lifted the tennis ball off the bed today on his own. He follows

---

commands, but not regularly. I wish there was a clear order for the staff to get him into the cardiac chair every day. He wakes up a little when he sits in that chair, but there is no set schedule. It appears to be up to the nurses and therapists, and some do it, and some do not. I have also been warned by our new friends, the Fritz family, not to let him sit in that chair for more than an hour per day because he can develop bedsores. Bedsores are a real demon to fight now. I admit I never understood how dangerous they could be, some even require surgery. I have also heard that some rehabs will refuse to take a patient if they have existing bedsores. Could you imagine if we get Dylan that far and a bedsore stops us? I will not let that happen.

Regarding our friends, some, more than others, have a personal experience with this type of tragedy. The Fritz family has really helped us in the last few days. We didn't know these people prior to Dylan's accident, but they contacted us through a mutual friend when they heard about Dylan. Their son, Ashton, suffered a spinal injury a few years ago and they were also covered by Kaiser. They were able to get their son to the Craig Hospital in Boulder, Colorado. Craig Hospital is highly ranked in the world of TBIs and spinal injuries and has a special program just for teenage patients. It is the only program like that in the world. They warned us that Kaiser would resist sending Dylan there because it is very expensive. They ended up giving us a road map on how to navigate Kaiser, to get Dylan the best treatment. They shared their story and what they had done. They told us that insurance companies hate three things: 1) spending money, 2) lawsuits, and 3) bad press. To get Kaiser to spend money on our son, we would have to show our willingness and ability to do two and three. Finally, something I can sink my teeth into. I am more than willing to fight; we all are.

First, Dylan must be declared "ready" for a post-acute rehab facility. A post-acute facility is what I would call an actual rehab, as opposed to sub-acute, which is more of a nursing home. If he is not ready for a post-acute facility, then he will likely go to the sub-acute facility, a nursing home. We are now hearing horror stories about teenagers in these facilities. We cannot let that happen. I let the patient coordinator know we would be asking for Craig Hospital when the time came, and she said she has never heard of it. The patient coordinator was a short lady who seemed nice enough. She told me she used to be a nurse and she would help steer the way for me to get Dylan to the best care possible for him. She was our contact and would meet with me several times per week.

Yesterday, Gabby arranged for two of Dylan's friends, Lucas and Alex, to have access to see him. We are worried about COVID, but we can also see how Dylan needs the stimulation. Stimulation from friends is much different than stimulation from parents and siblings. US Air Force ROTC has really sharpened Gabby's leadership skills. She not only found a way to get the hospital administration to let the friends in, but she also quizzed the boys for any symptoms of COVID and made them promise to keep their masks on and follow the hospital's rules. This was our choice to assume the COVID risk and we were willing to gamble a little. We really think these types of visits could help wake Dylan up. If Dylan did have to go to sub-acute, then we were insisting that he go to a place that allowed visitors. We would accept going back to just me and Cindy, but we had to be able to be with him twenty-four hours a day. I relayed this to the patient coordinator, but she felt it would be very difficult to find such a place. We instinctively knew Dylan would not get any better if we were not with him, so this was a possible looming battle.

JUNE 20, 2020 – THIRTY-NINE DAYS SINCE THE ACCIDENT.

It is now eight days until Dylan turns eighteen. Dylan is still not ready for post-acute rehab, but we have launched our offensive arguments to make sure he gets to Craig Hospital when the time is right. We started an online petition urging Kaiser to send Dylan to Craig Hospital's one-of-a-kind treatment program. The petition has over 2,000 signatures already and, Arik Armstead, from the San Francisco 49ers, just sent the link out on his Instagram account so we knew the number of signatures would continue to grow. Matthew, who is still in law school, is researching how the appeal process works if Kaiser says no. He has some wonderful professors who have been assisting him. Erica is writing a summary of Dylan's life story, which we will include with any formal appeal we file. My sister is researching statistics comparing Craig Hospital to Kaiser facilities to show where the best treatment for Dylan truly exists. We have also contacted an admissions specialist for Craig Hospital and are sending them some of Dylan's medical records so they can be prepared to accept him.

We wanted to make the public aware of Dylan's fight, so I reached out via Twitter to Cameron Salerno. I believe he was an unpaid intern at the *Sac Bee* at the time who covered high school sports, including football. He had tweeted out some coverage about Dylan over the past few months. Cameron, who was not much older than Dylan, responded immediately and said he was aware of Dylan's accident, and he had already passed along news of the petition. Cameron inquired with the *Sac Bee* and ended up being assigned to write the article himself. Cameron called and spoke with Erica and I and did some follow-up research before writing a very nice article, which appeared in the sports section a few days later. Cameron's family is also involved with local high school sports, and they do a lot of photography at sporting events. They had a database of photos of Dylan and supplied the senior night photo with all of us to be used with the article. They also gave us a bunch of other photos they had taken, including some of Dylan carrying the Folsom flag onto the field before the game, an honor which showed how much his teammates respected him.

I previously mentioned we were all waiting for something constructive to do, everyone was just begging for an assignment. I also keep reminding the patient coordinator that we will not accept a sub-acute facility that does not allow visitors. I believe the doctors, nurses, and administrative workers we speak to do understand why we are doing this, but ultimately, they do not make the decisions. We are Dylan's best therapy and best allies. If he is awake, we are stimulating him, no matter which one of us is in the room. Ultimately, it is still Cindy or myself eighty percent of the time right now. Dylan would not be this far along without us, and he will only get the best care if we push for it.

Today, Dylan sat in the cardiac chair and played a little tug of war with me over a piece of gauze. I have video of it that I texted out in our group threads. This was a good day! Before I came in, Lucas had been in for another visit. They only allow one visitor at a time, so I waited in the lobby until Lucas was finished. When he met me in the lobby, I could see Lucas was emotional, so that made me emotional. I told Lucas that everything will be ok, and that by all rights, Dylan should have died. So, we are blessed to have this opportunity with him. Dylan is improving a little bit at a time, so we all just need to keep going. We must be thankful for the opportunity and be strong for Dylan. Is it weird that it is easier for me to be strong for others than for myself? Lucas told me he played a song for Dylan before he left and it was a song they used to jam to, so it made him sad. When I got up to the room, the nurse told me that Lucas' visit had really perked Dylan up. His eyes were wide open, his arms were moving, and she even thinks Dylan may have smiled. One of my biggest wishes is for Dylan to be able to smile. God is good.

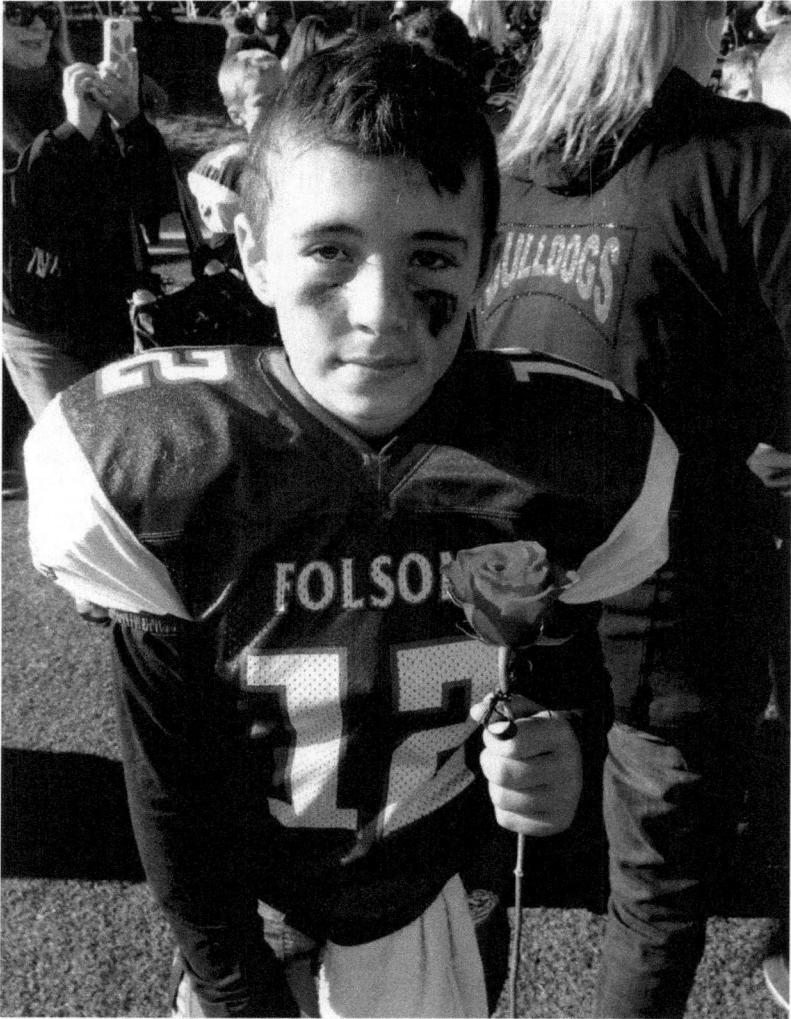

Dylan with a rose for his Mom during his first year of football.

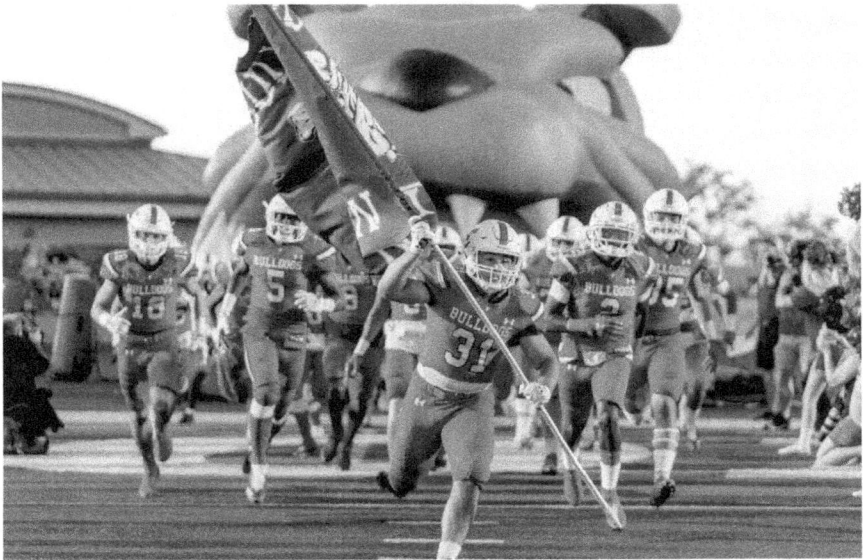
Dylan (31) leading the team onto the field during his senior year.

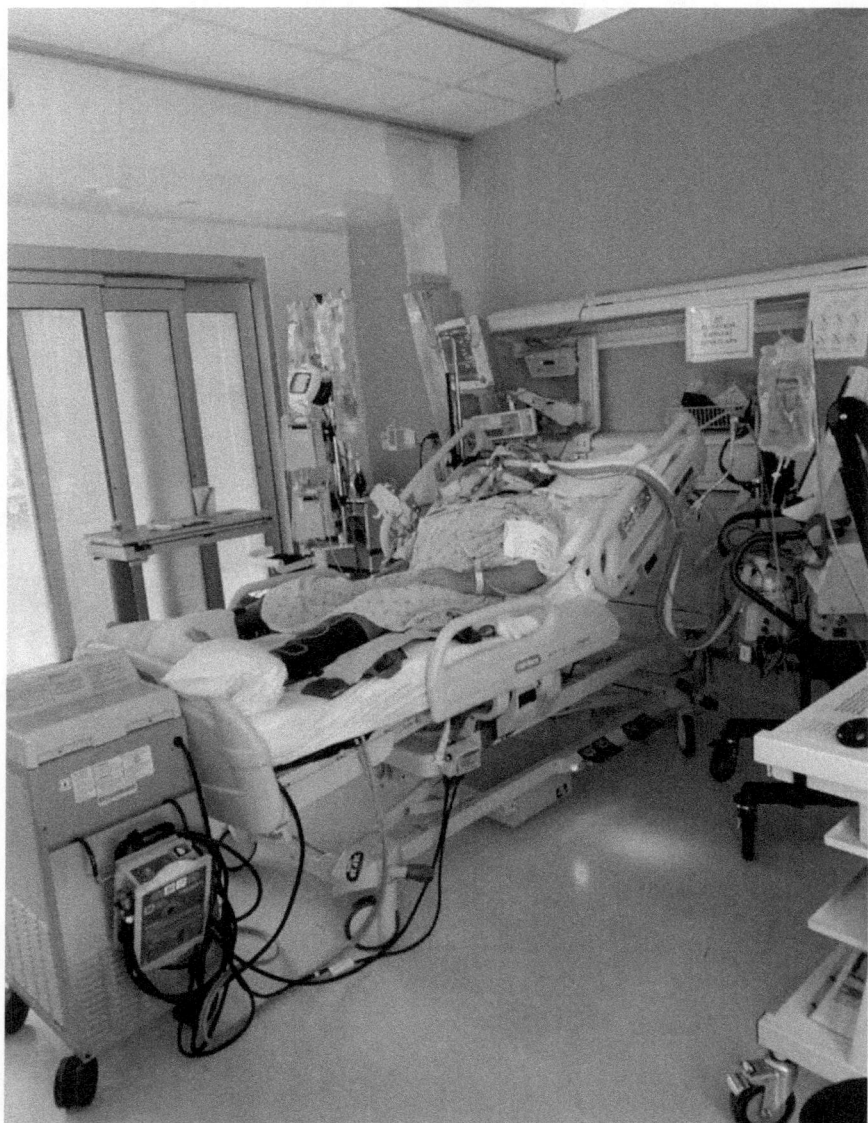

Dylan at UC Davis Medical Center 18 days after the accident.

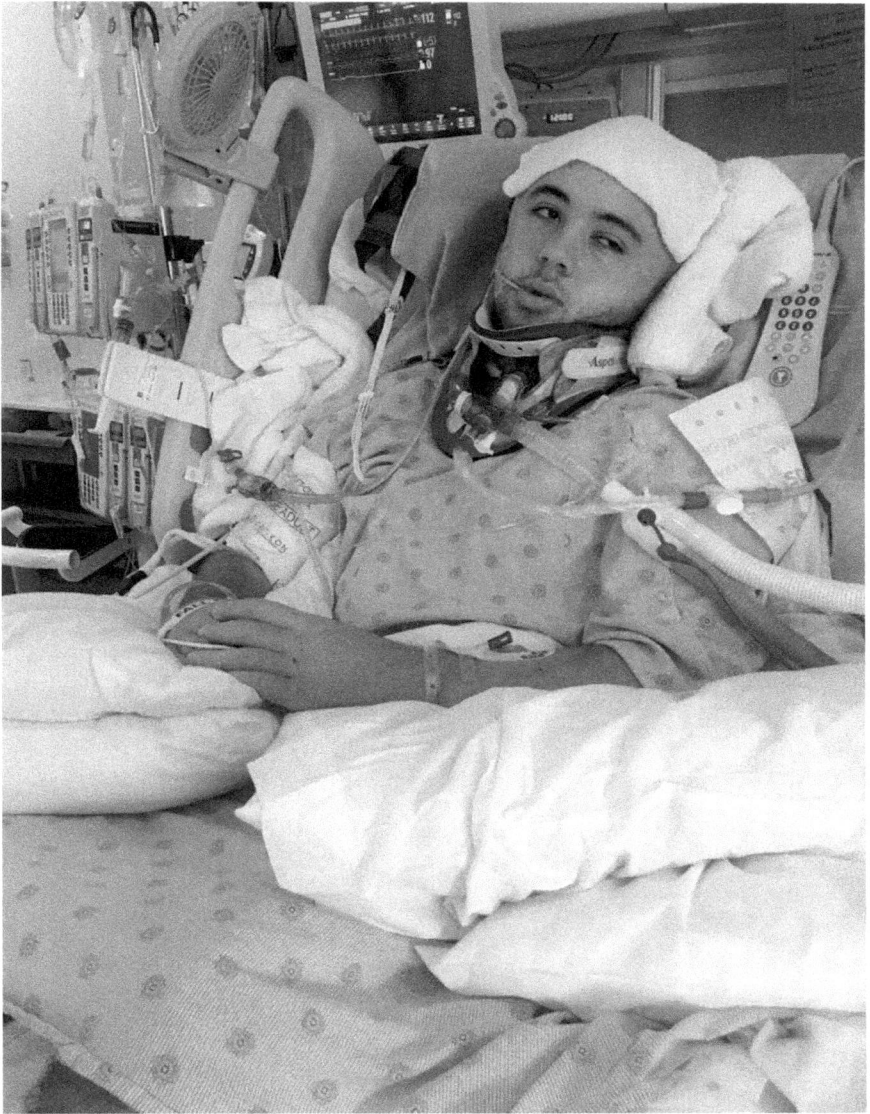

June 5, 2020. A rare moment with open eyes.

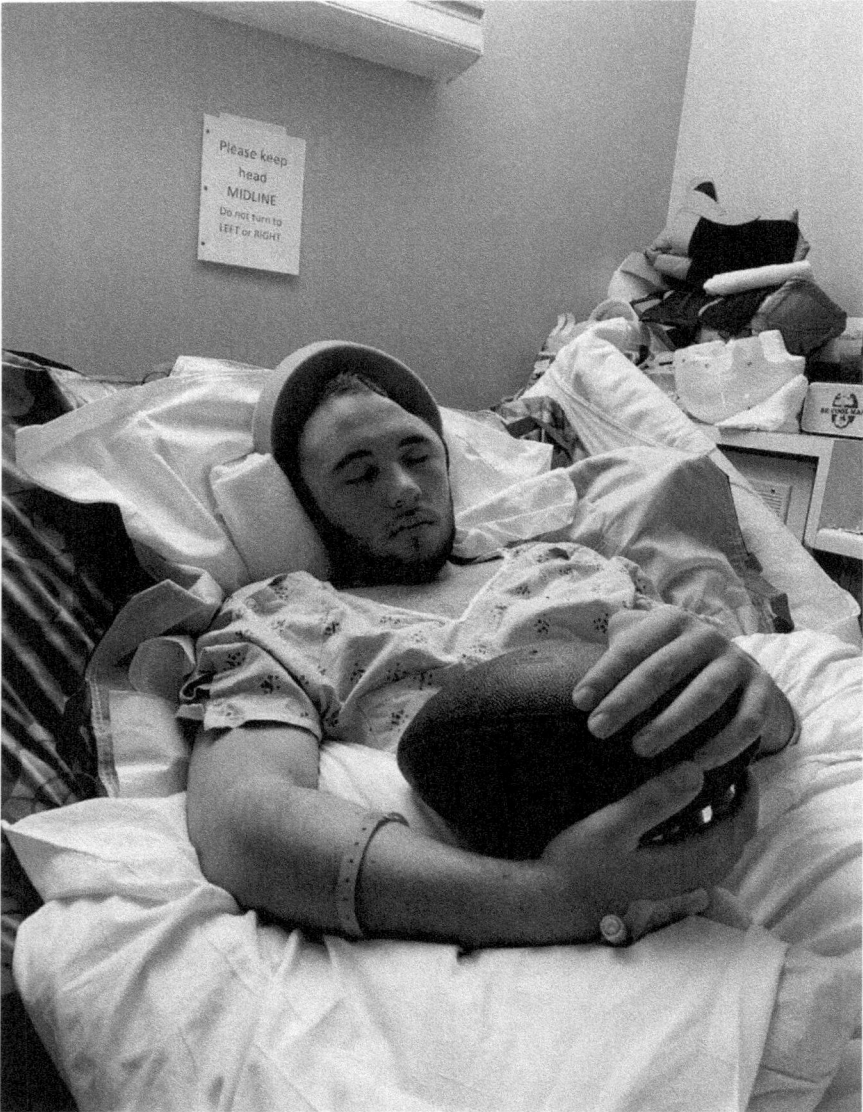

The moment he touched a football he knew what to do with it.

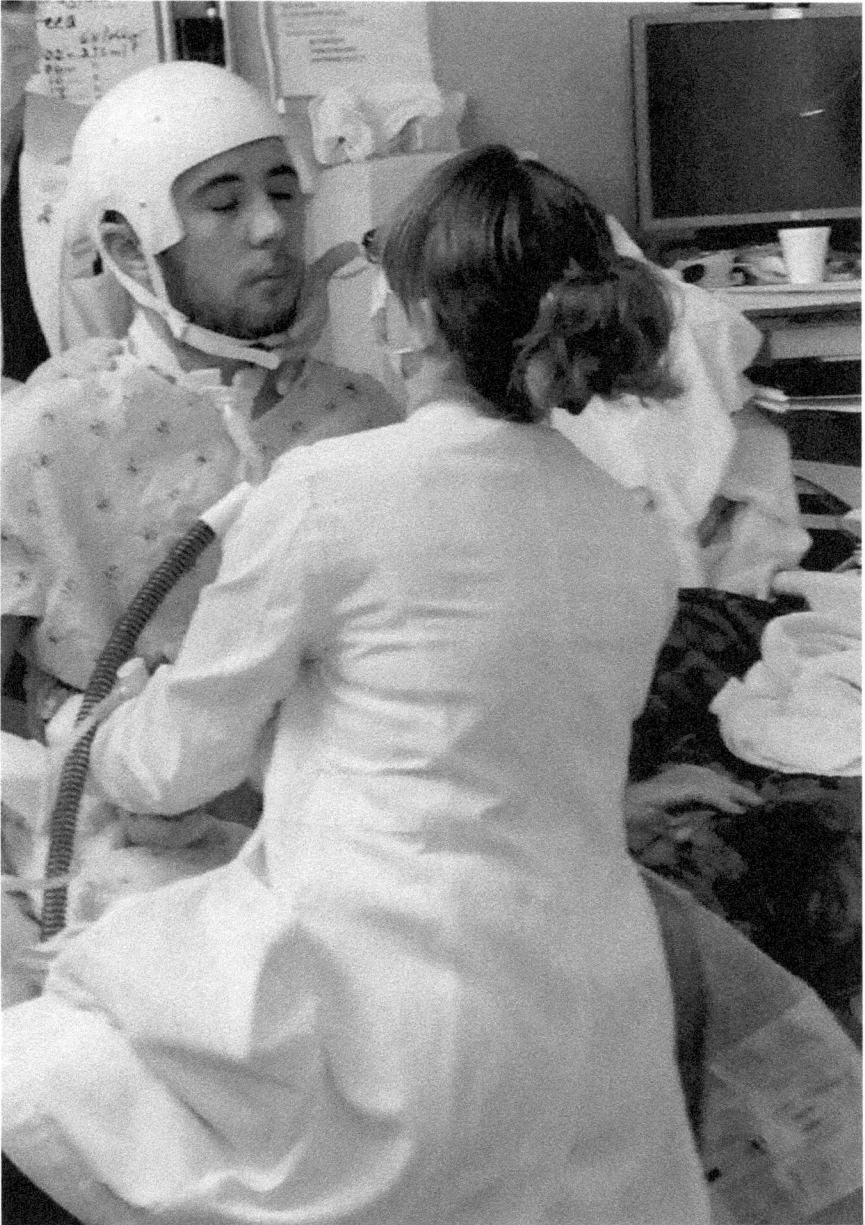

Dylan's 18th Birthday. Therapists from Kaiser Hospital – Morse try to get him to sit up.

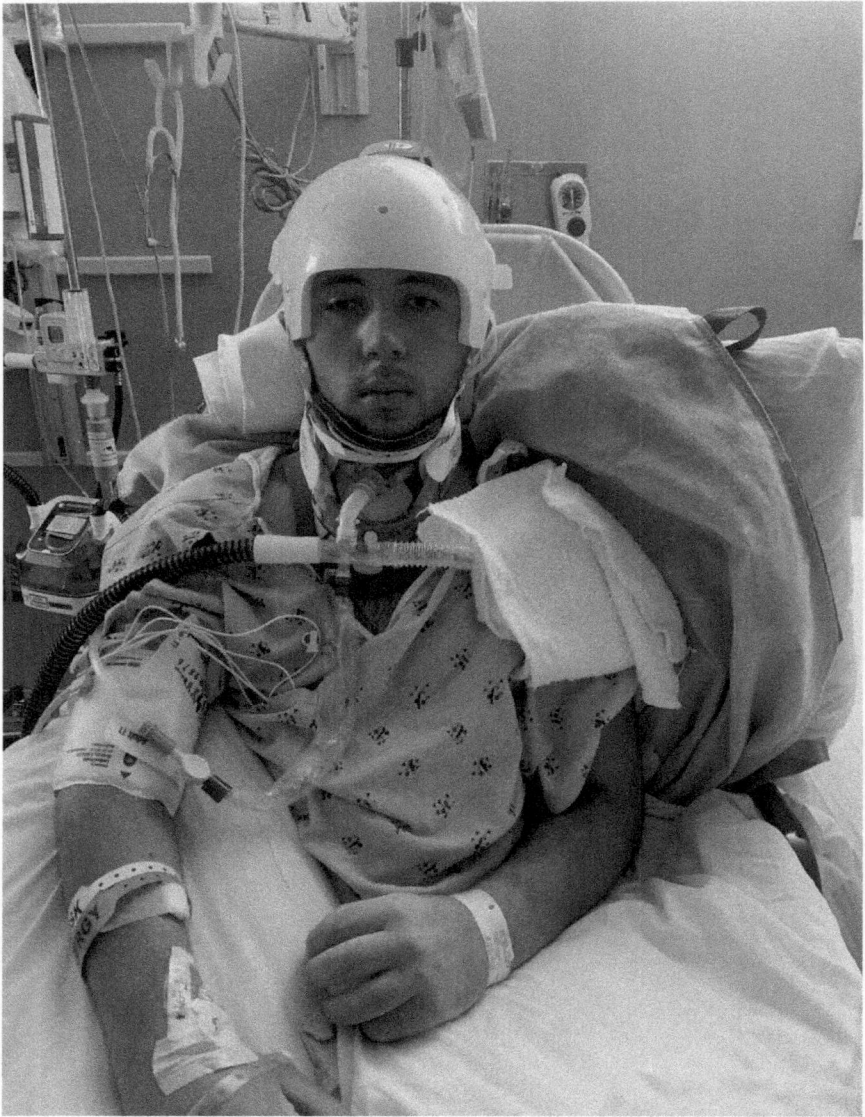

Sitting in the Cardiac Chair often helped to wake him.

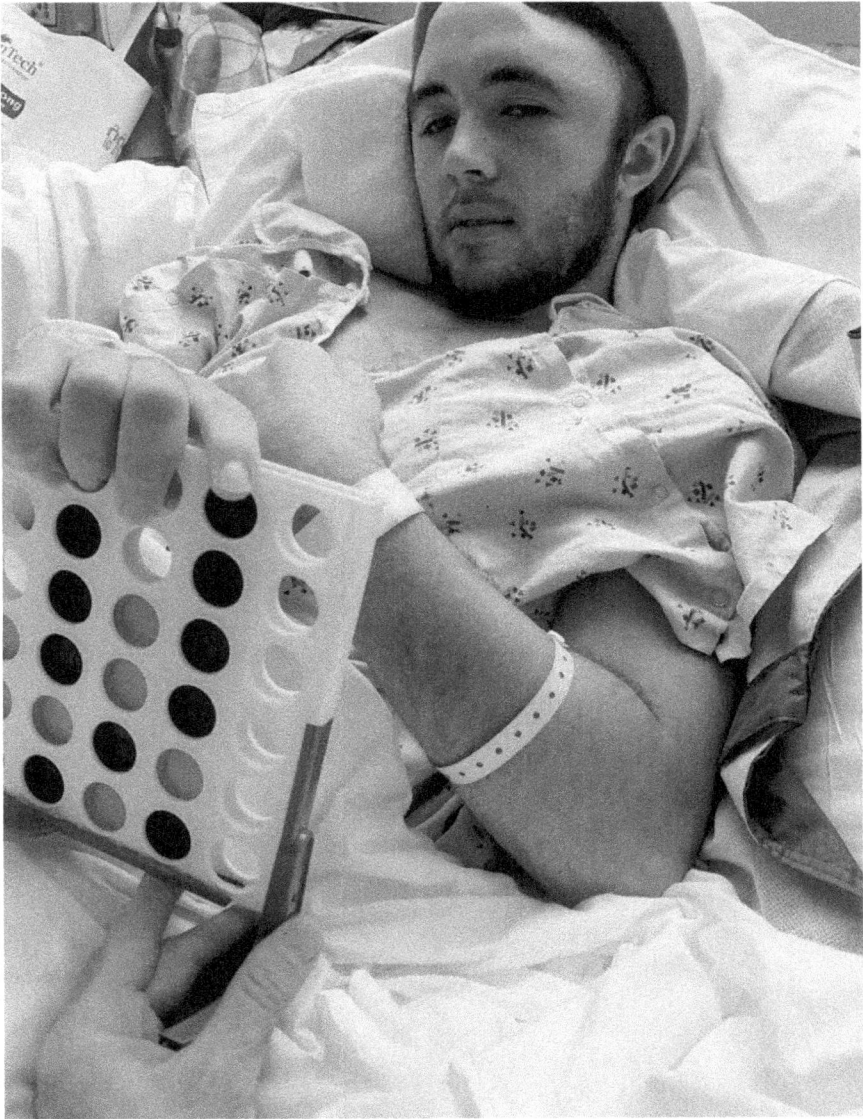

Beating Dad in Connect Four.

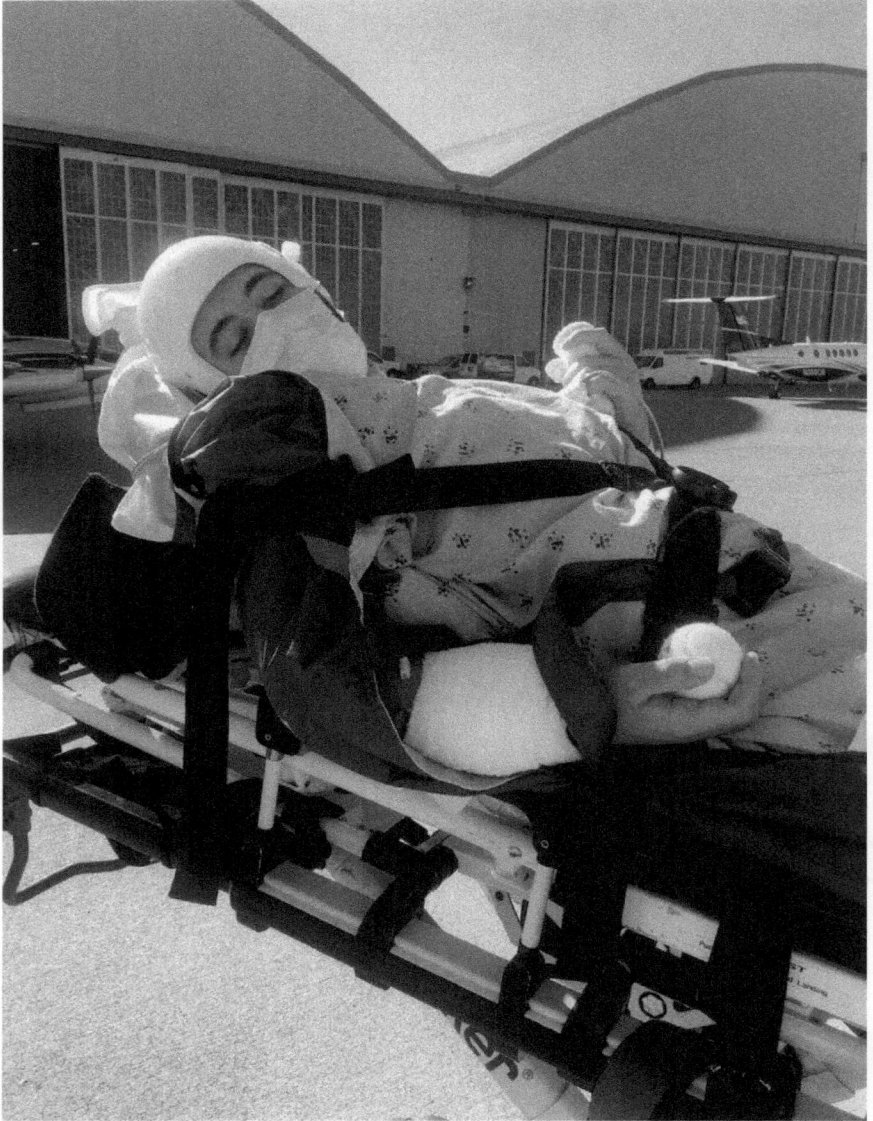

July 22, 2020, 0n his way to Craig Hospital

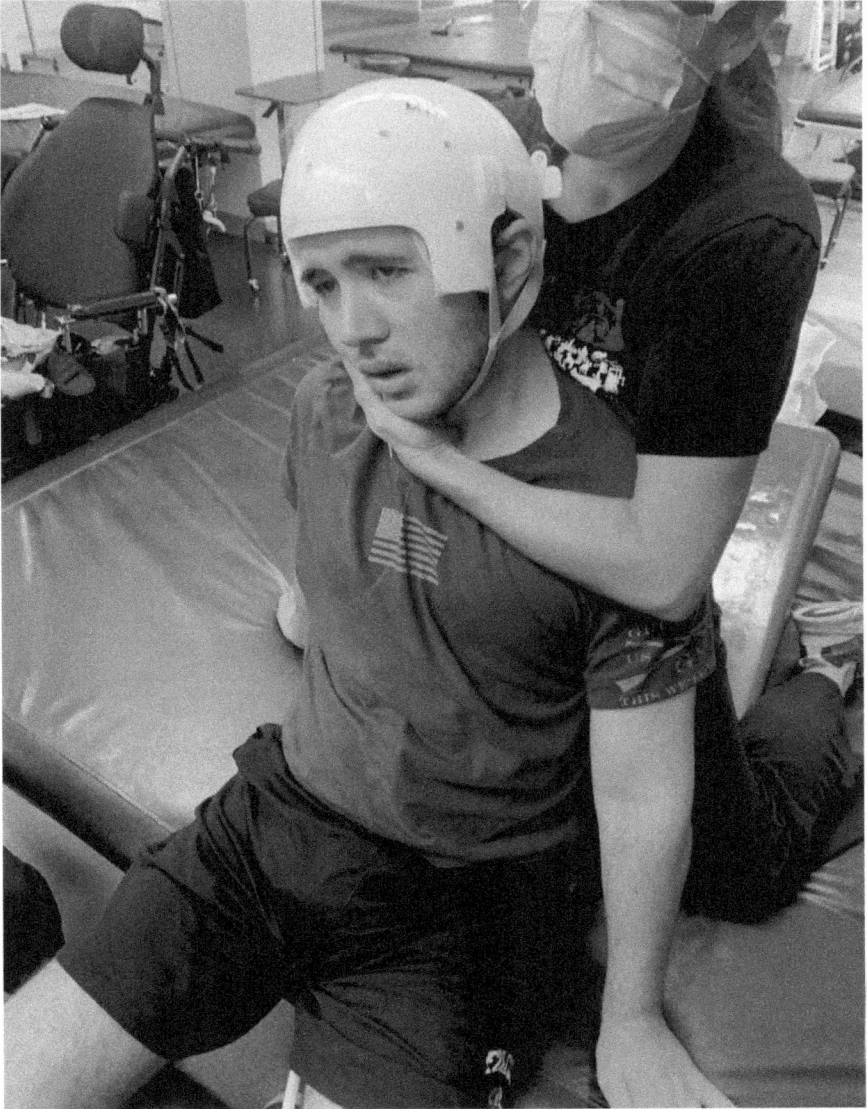

Therapy can be painful

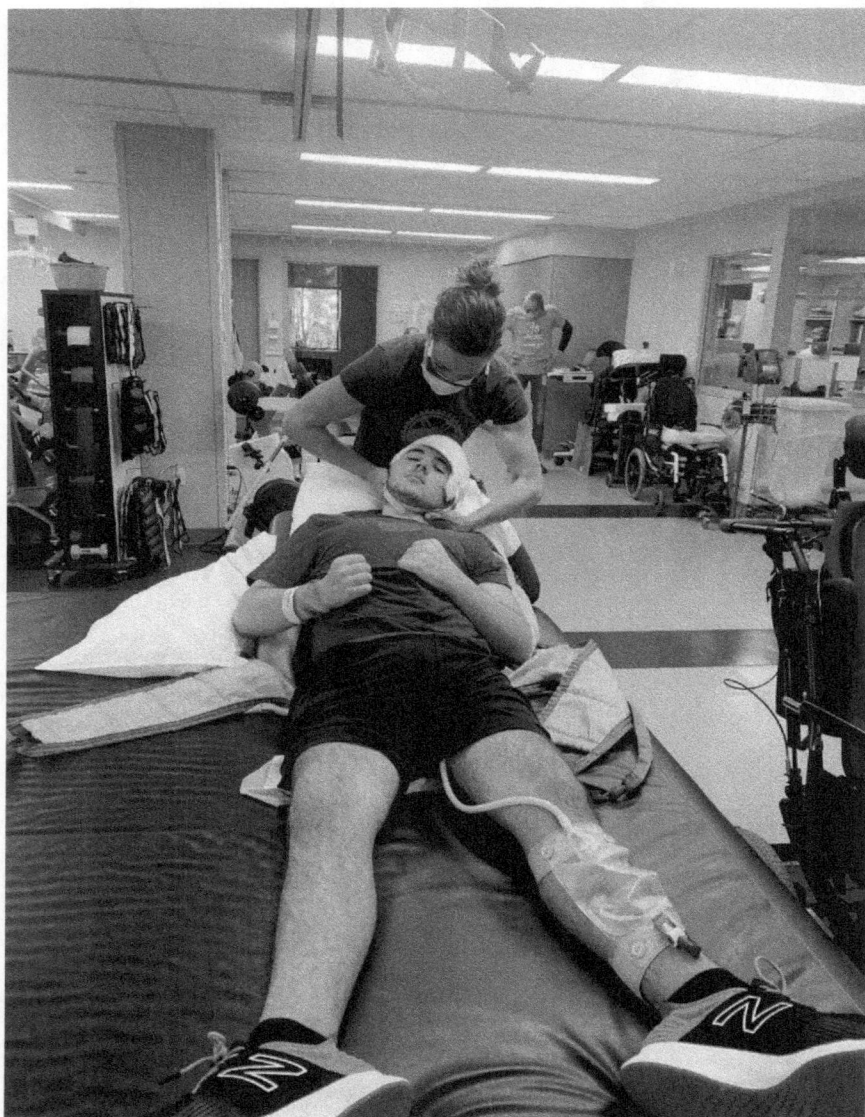

Keeping his muscles loose.

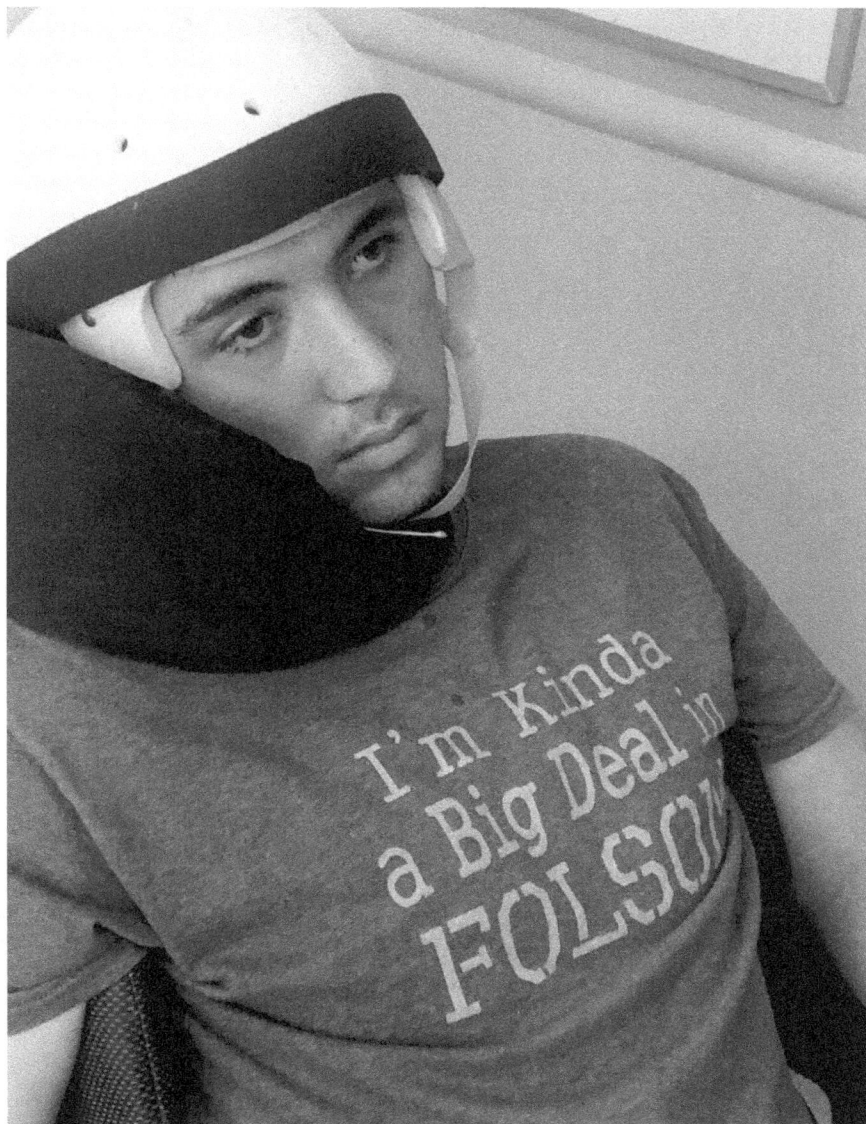

Headband and neck pillow to hold his head up.

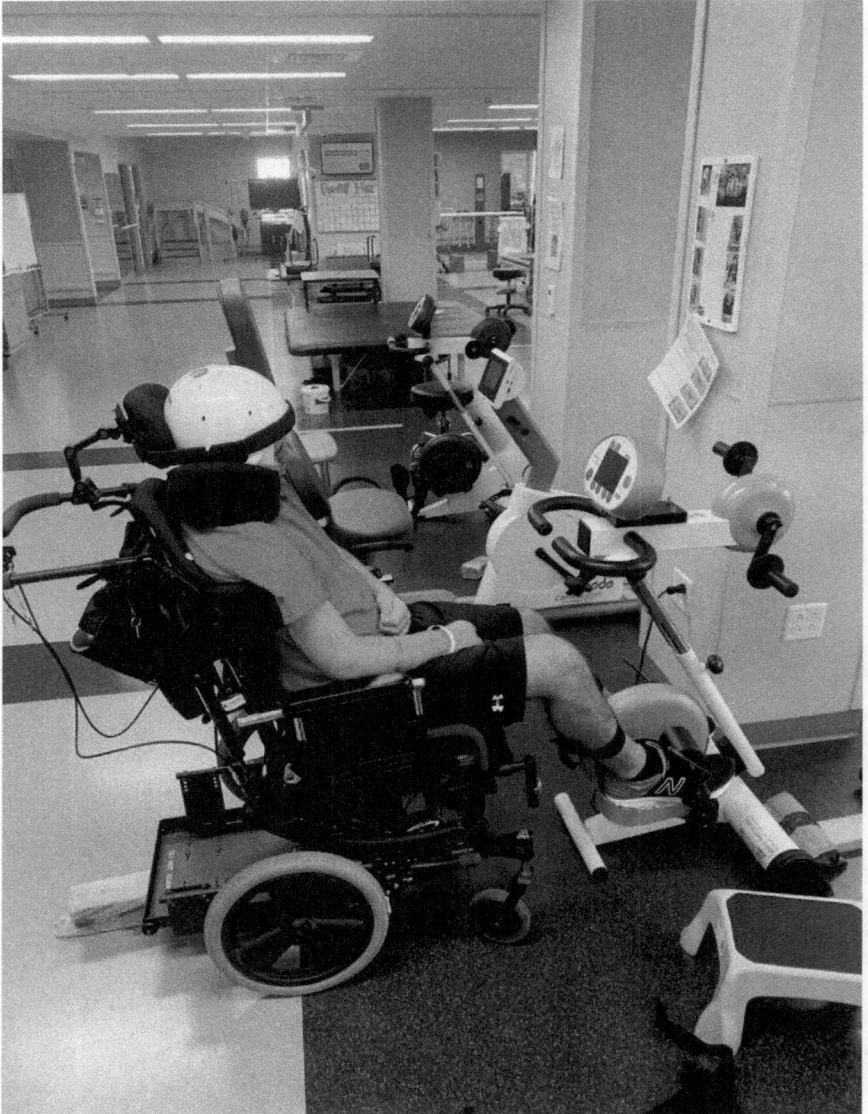

The exercise bike that could pedal for him if necessary.

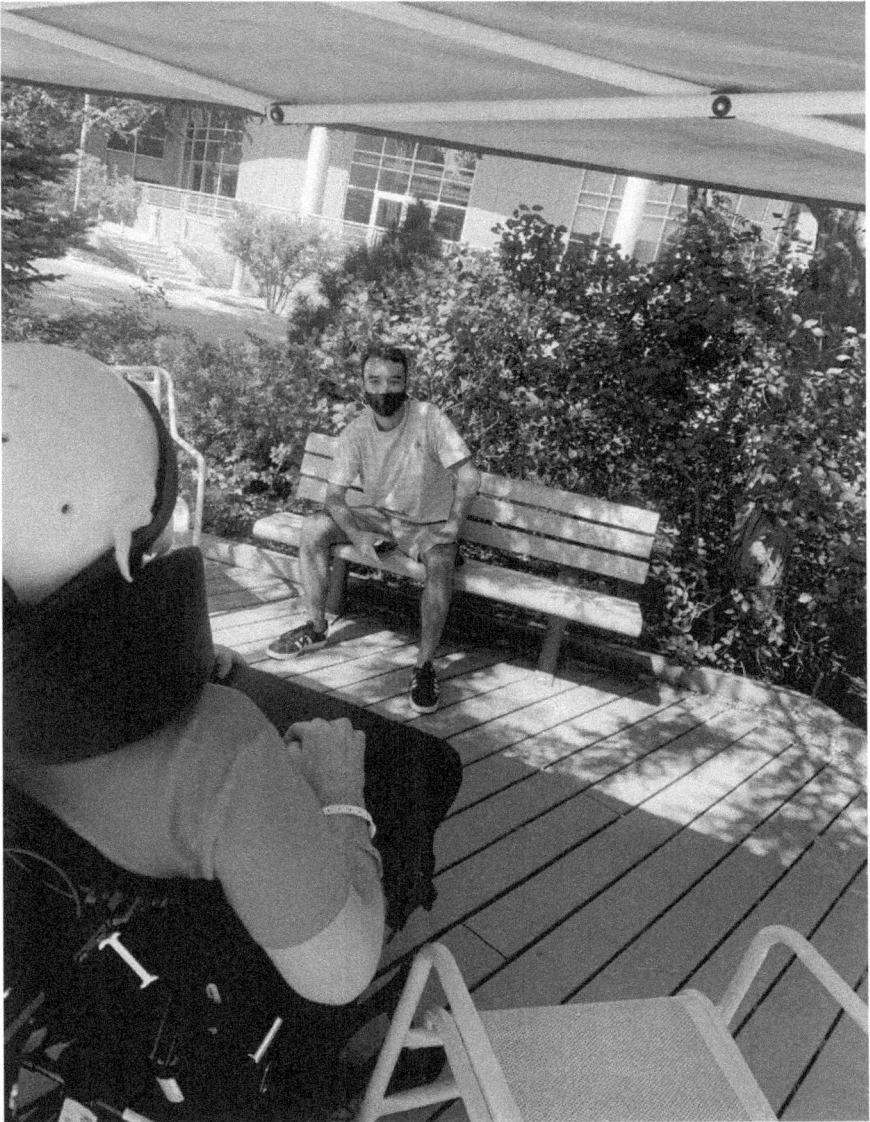

Matthew visiting Dylan in the garden at Craig Hosital.

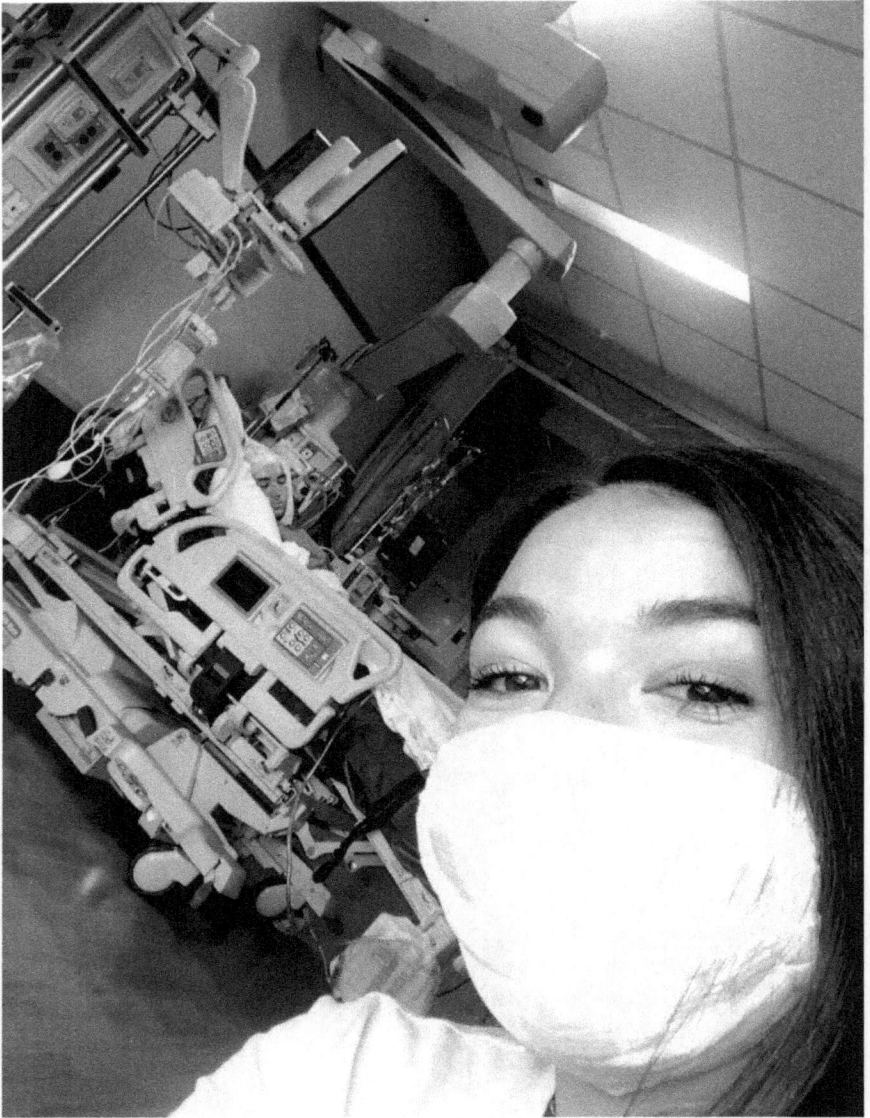

Gabby with Dylan at St. Joseph's Hospital.

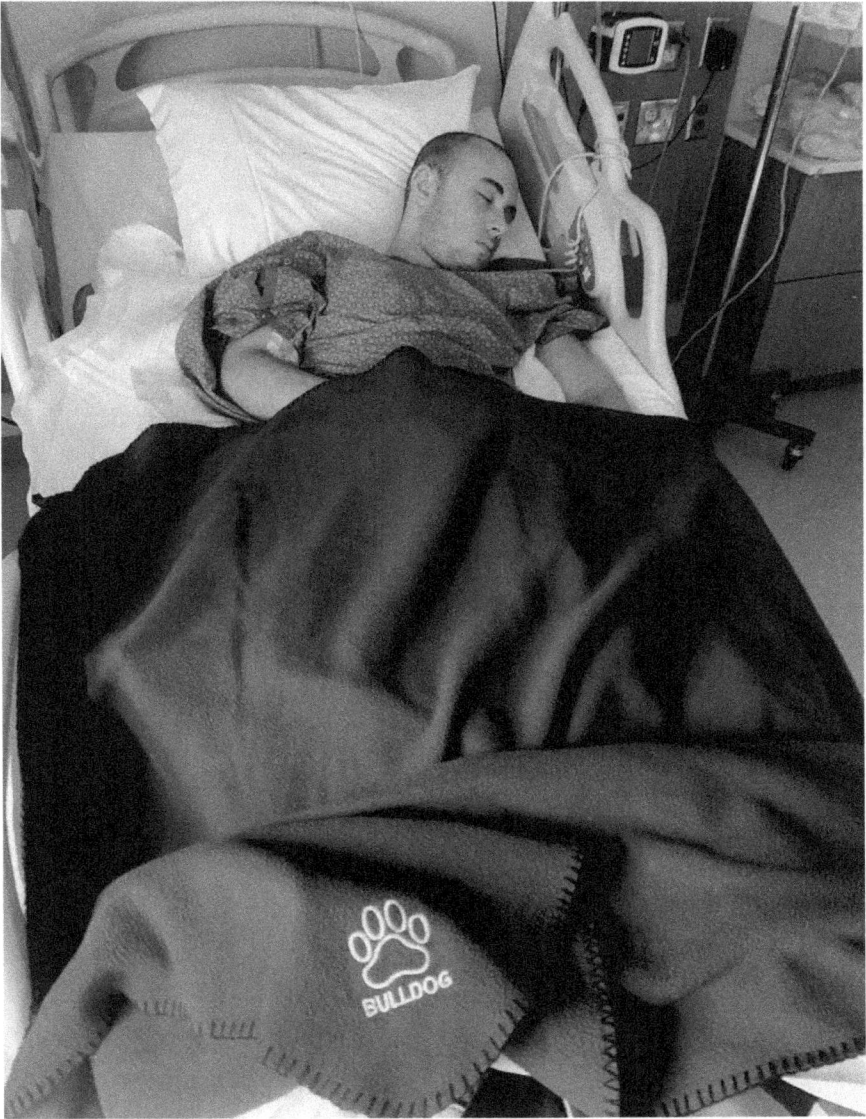

Dylan with his new skull plates in place.

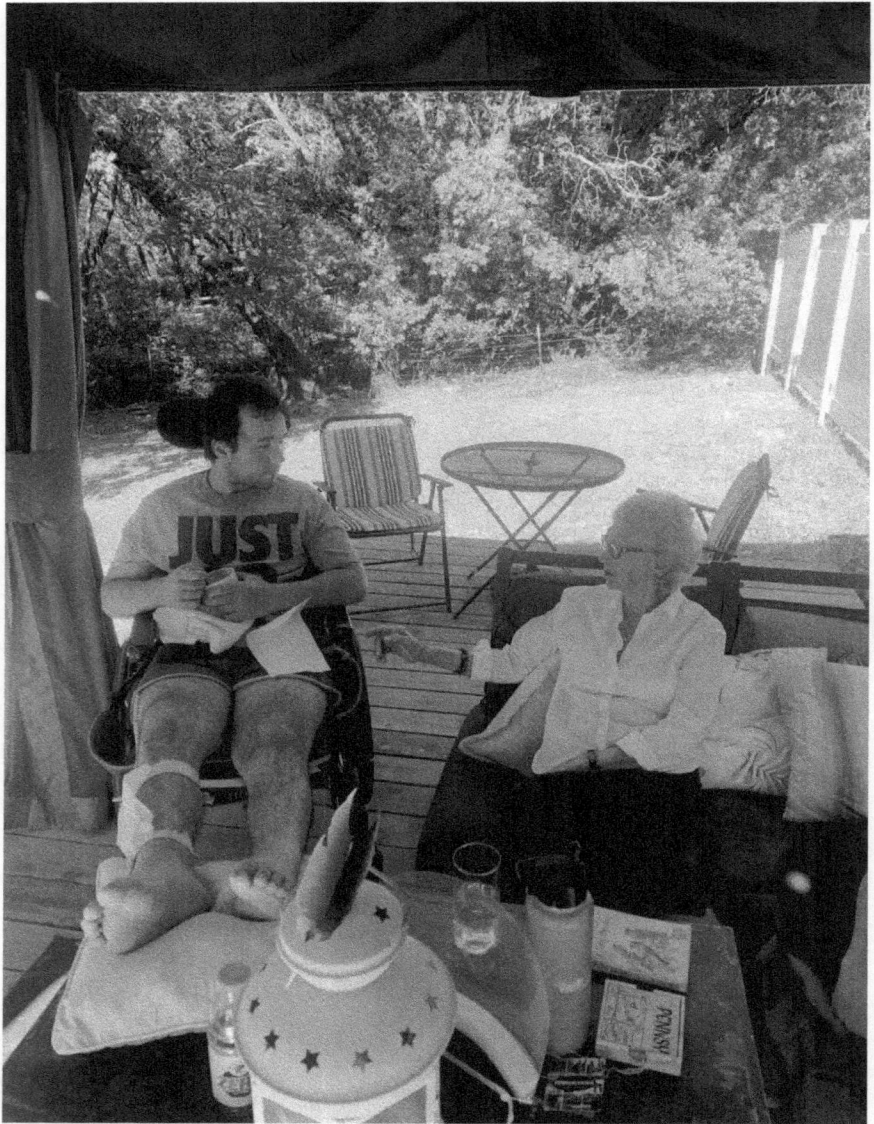

May 2021. Dylan visiting with his grandmother.

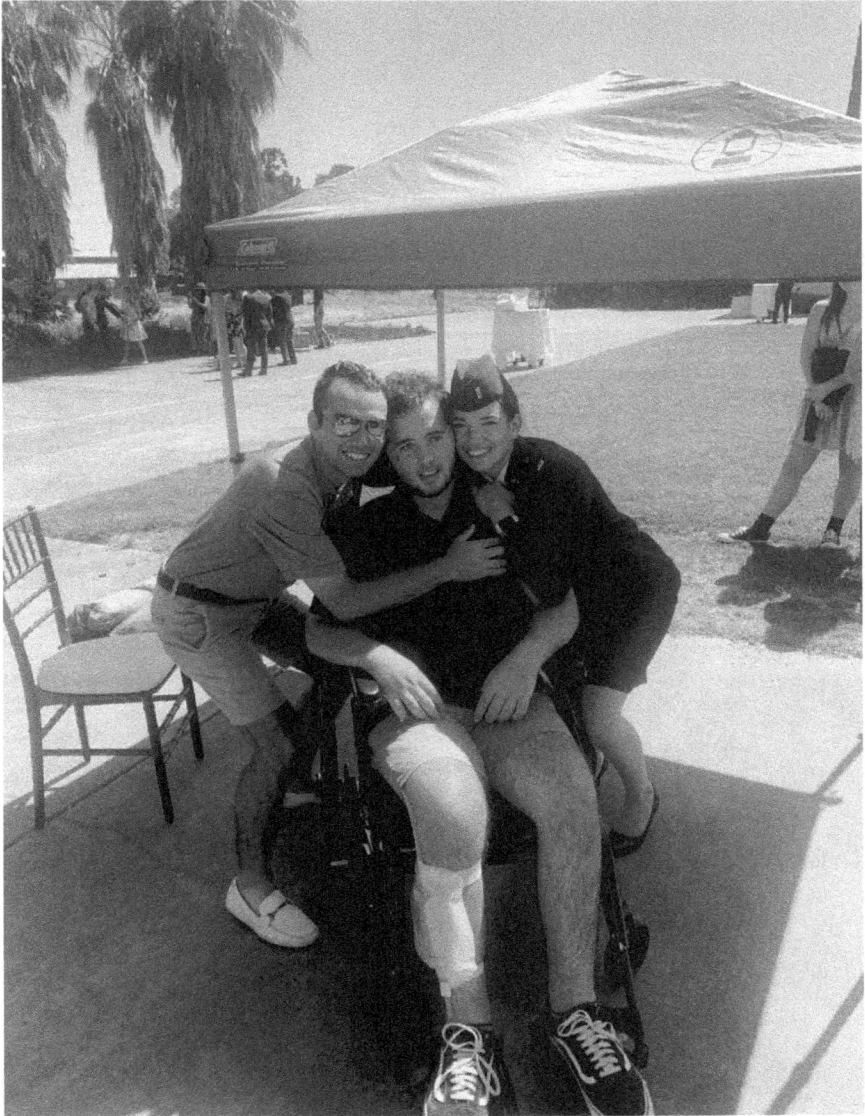

Matthew, Gabby and Dylan.

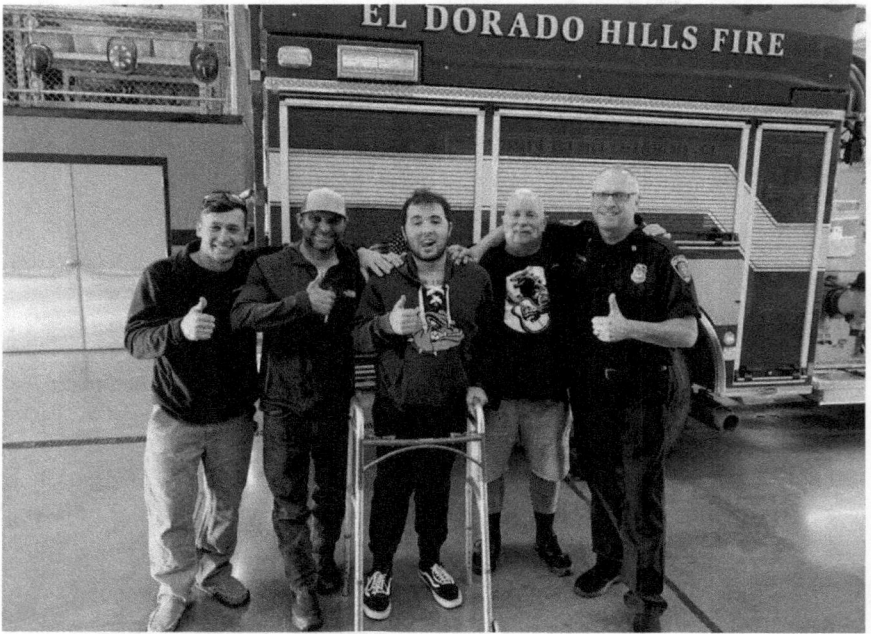

Dylan got to meet and thank the heroes who gave him a chance.

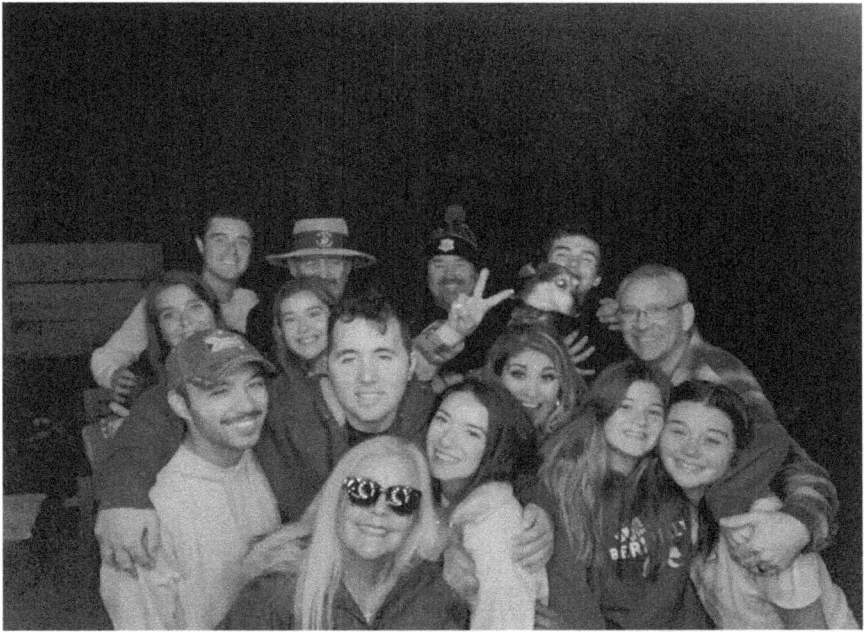

Thanksgiving 2021. A real reason to be thankful.

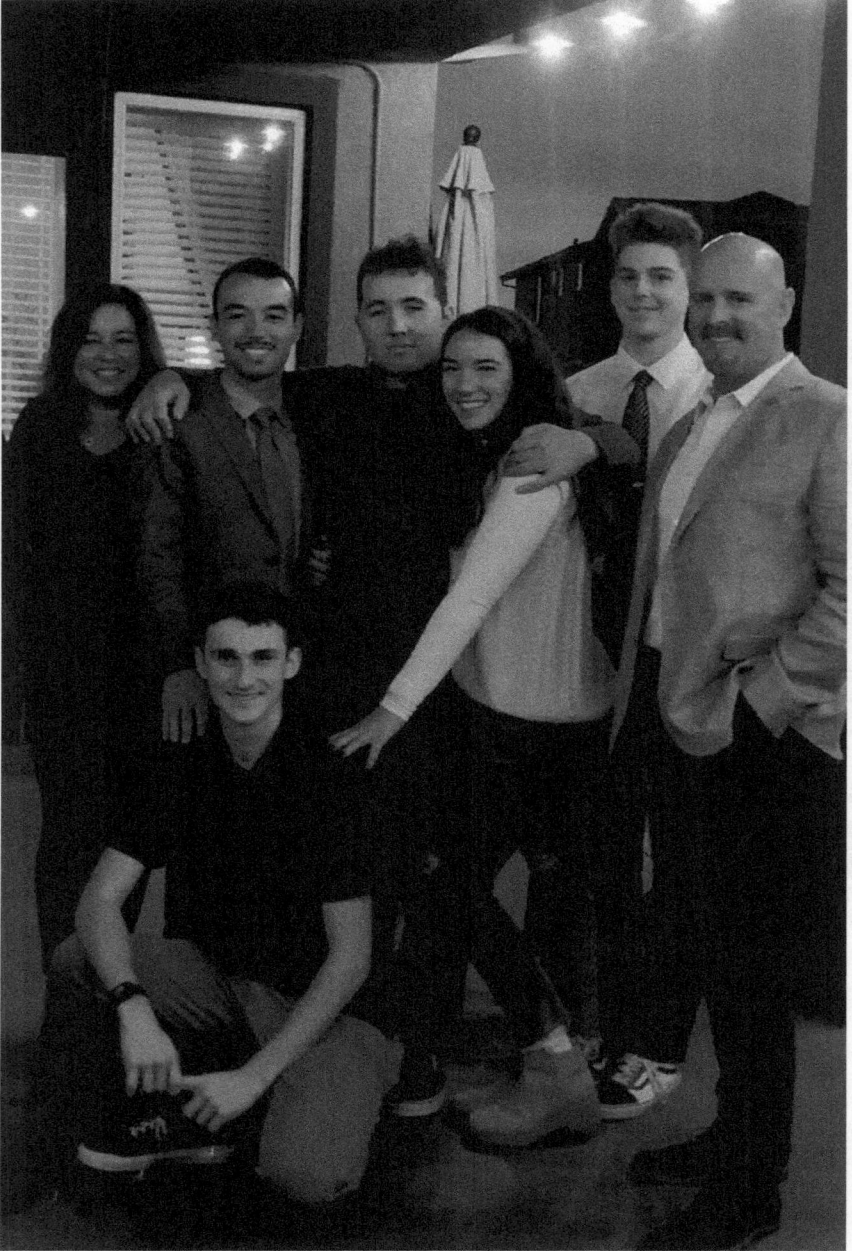

Cindy, Pablo, Matthew, Gabby, Zach and Josh with Dylan.

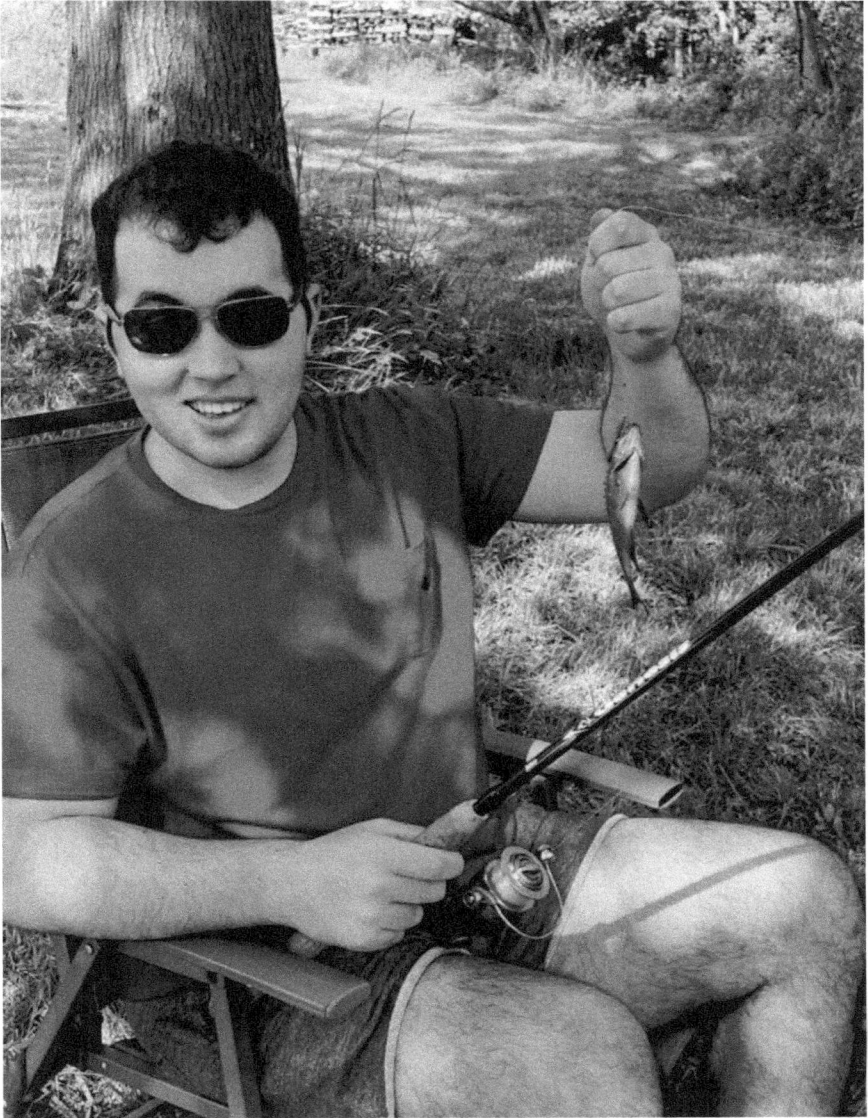

Any fish is a good fish when it is an answered prayer!

Chapter 7

FOLLOWING SIMPLE COMMANDS

JUNE 23, 2020 – FORTY-TWO DAYS SINCE THE ACCIDENT.

Yesterday at eleven a.m., Dylan woke up and out of the blue, he began tracking me with his eyes. Tracking simply means he followed me with his eyes as I walked around his room. It was the most beautiful and amazing thing I had seen in a long time. I wanted to cry tears of joy, but I also felt that permeable fear of what if this is it, or what if he doesn't wake up any further? Being in the hospital eight or more hours per day means that I hear every doctor's worst-case scenario. Now, they seem to be focusing on who will care for Dylan at home. Do you have a single-story home, a handicapped accessible shower, etc.? I had to fight myself to just enjoy this moment. Dylan's eyes are open, and he is tracking me!

Later we played some thumb wars, and I taught him a handshake. This is an incredible day, and we are only six weeks in; we have a long, long way to go, and the possibilities are almost endless. We are preparing for a fight with Kaiser over getting Dylan to Craig Hospital. I have been talking to admissions at Craig Hospital and they are telling me Dylan is almost ready for post-acute. I truly believe that the best chance for Dylan to have a good life is through Craig Hospital. I will fight with all my heart to get him there. It will likely mean I will go weeks at a time without seeing him, but I know he will be in the best hands. I have heard that the recovery in the first few months is very important. We only get one shot at doing what is best for him and we live with that for the rest of our lives.

JUNE 24, 2020 – FORTY-THREE DAYS SINCE THE ACCIDENT.

Kaiser has decided that Dylan is ready for a post-acute facility, and they issued a letter saying he is going to their San Jose facility, a good facility. I want to be clear that we never meant to imply that the Kaiser facilities were not adequate. They are well-respected, but they do lack the specific program designed for teenagers with traumatic brain injuries that Craig Hospital offers. Why not give Dylan his best possible chance? I spoke with the patient coordinator and told her again that we wanted Craig Hospital. She looked me in the eye and replied, **"NO!"** I didn't handle that well. I could feel the rage build up inside me. As the tears came to my eyes, I managed to spit out the words, "How dare you! How dare you flippantly say no to what my son needs." I am not proud of it, but I believe a few F-bombs may have spilled out in my next few sentences. I could see she was taken aback by my reaction and maybe a little scared. I didn't mean for that, but if she thinks she is going to say a dismissive "NO" to my face and that is the end of it, then she has another thing coming.

As my wife likes to point out, I was raised in the Philadelphia area. I don't react well to things I feel negatively impact my family members. We had already had an article published about Dylan's story in the local paper, *The Sacramento Bee.* I told the patient coordinator we were going to appeal Kaiser's decision legally and go back to the paper so the community will be aware. The next morning my cell phone rang, and it was the ombudsman from Kaiser. My understanding is that the ombudsman is like an unofficial go-between, a way to begin a dialogue, for senior management. It is very wise for an organization like Kaiser to have an ombudsman. She said she represents the higher-ups in the organization, and she would like to know what our wishes are for Dylan and why. I explained our feelings to her and told her we know Kaiser has sent teenagers to Craig Hospital before. We will accept nothing less than Dylan going to Craig Hospital and we will appeal any decision which doesn't send him there. We will also make sure the entire community supporting Dylan knows about the fight.

The next day I got a new letter—Dylan was going to Craig Hospital. Thank you, God, for sending us the Fritz family! This would have been a much more drawn-out fight without their excellent advice. This gives Dylan his best chance. This is all I can ask for from the insurance company. When I saw the patient coordinator again, she was extremely pleasant. Almost relieved, I think. My belief is that she was likely told to tell us no and to be firm. She was just the unfortunate point person. She did say we would likely have to pay for a medical flight to get Dylan to Colorado, but at that point I didn't care. As it turns out she was wrong and one flight per accident was covered by insurance. I immediately notified Craig Hospital and they said they will begin working with Kaiser to determine when it is best to transfer him. Depending on the COVID policy at Craig Hospital, we will have to wait and see who goes with Dylan. I am less worried about that; I mean, one fight at a time, right? I know someone will be by his side and I know he will be getting the best care he can get. Most of the work there will be done by therapists, not family. So far, we have been the ones pushing him. Now, we just need to keep him from getting any bedsores or COVID and wait for the transfer date.

In another positive development, Dylan also had the moisturizing machine removed from his trach. When the speech therapist came in and plugged his trach hole, he was able to say something—"hello"— was the first word I heard from him since the accident. It was low and scratchy, but I heard it! I remember my fears about the trach going in at UC Davis. I was so scared that it was never coming out. Tears of joy!

JUNE 28, 2020 – FORTY-SEVEN DAYS SINCE THE ACCIDENT.

Dylan's birthday! I know it is not the eighteenth birthday any kid would want but we can't change that now. We brought in some cookies for the nurses and a few of them came into Dylan's room and sang "Happy Birthday" to him. He is here for it and making progress. Last night, Cindy sent out a video of Dylan holding his left arm in the air and then raising and lowering it on command. I have not seen him do that before, I believe that is what they mean by "follows simple commands." When I got to the hospital, I had Dylan repeat the movement for my mom while she FaceTimed us for his birthday. My brother FaceTimed us later and at the end of that call, I got Dylan to stick his tongue out at him. We all got a great big laugh at that one. My brother saw me at an extremely low point, so it is good he got to see some of this now. Cindy had also gotten video of Dylan putting his fingers up and down as she counted. It has been an incredible few days! This is the best I have felt in a long time. It is amazing the people who continue to reach out. Yesterday I spoke with a mother from Seattle whose son had a TBI from a longboard accident just like Dylan. She said they got a similar dire report from the neurologist and just under a year later, their son jokes, walks, talks, and is learning to read. She told me that no one can tell me where Dylan will end up, because no one knows. For the first time I am allowing myself to feel real hope that Dylan may yet laugh and fish with me again. I can live with that.

JULY 1, 2020 – FIFTY DAYS SINCE THE ACCIDENT.

Today was another awesome day! Gabby sent out a video of Dylan mouthing her name and one of him mouthing "I love you." The "I love you" made everyone who saw it cry. When I took my shift at the hospital, I brought a football with me. When I handed it to Dylan, he held the football correctly with the three points of contact that is taught to running backs. Dylan moved his arm back and forth like he was running with it. After that, I even got him to try to throw a tennis ball. It didn't really go anywhere but at least he tried. Later, Dylan was very alert and as I spoke with him, he really seemed to understand what I was saying. I asked him if he knew what happened to him and he raised his hand a little and seemed to point to his head. I explained all the surgeries he had, and how far he has come, and how great he is doing. I explained how we got him into Craig Hospital, which is the best place in the world for his injury. I told him he has a lot of hard work ahead of him, but we will be with him every step of the way. I made sure to point out that he is already an inspiration to a lot of people. I also told him that people from all over the world—friends, family, and strangers—are praying for him. I can hardly believe I am sitting here doing this right now. I don't want it to end but I know that it will. He gets tired very easy. It is so nice to have some interaction with him. This really fueled my hope for the future. Dylan is completely off all oxygen and the trach should come out soon. God is great!

JULY 3, 2020 — FIFTY-TWO DAYS SINCE THE ACCIDENT.

When I got here this morning Dylan was sleeping. Around eight a.m. I noticed he was moving his arms, so I went to his bedside to say good morning. To my surprise, he opened his eyes, took a few seconds to focus on me, and then in a low, scratchy voice said, "Where is my mom?"

I was shocked and said, "What?"

He again said, "Where is my mom?"

I said, "She went home to rest, but I am here now, and she will be back later. *It's Dad!*"

He said, "Hi Dad!" and went back to sleep. That was it, a few seconds of interaction but the joy it brought me is almost indescribable. Dylan is in there.

At one p.m. they came in and removed his trach completely. I remember when they gave him the trach, how upset, and how scared I was that it may never come out. Well, it is out now. We are further down the road. My fears and stress from the time they were putting the trach in are gone, dissolved into the past. The hole in his throat may take up to a week to heal. My emotions may never fully heal, but that is ok, Dylan spoke a few words! Again, God is great!

Yesterday I met with four people from Craig Hospital. They were in Sacramento for a meeting and knew Dylan was on their admissions list, so they stopped by to say hello. Due to COVID, they could not get in to see Dylan, so we met in a park near the hospital. They gave me some brochures and answered a bunch of my questions. They told me Craig Hospital also has a strict COVID policy and currently limits visitation. I told them I am not a troublemaker. No one wants Dylan to avoid COVID more than me, but I am sure Craig Hospital understands the need for family stimulation of TBI patients. I only want what is best for Dylan. I want him as far back to normal as possible. Let's take this road to the best possible Amsterdam!

JULY 4, 2020 – FIFTY-THREE DAYS SINCE THE ACCIDENT.

When I think about whether I have guilty feelings, the simple answer is, yes, I have them sometimes. People like my former neighbor's daughter, Bill Fetterolf's son, or the stepson to my brother's ex-wife. All these young people whose parents never got to spend a little extra time with them. They never got to hear their voice again. Perhaps they were never given the chance to say goodbye. They never got to feel their child's kiss on their cheek again. My uncle Charlie died when I was around ten years old. I vividly recall all the sadness at the hospital and at the funeral service. I was in the room when they closed the casket for the last time and the sound of my grandmother crying is still with me. I don't have to close a casket; in that way I am truly blessed. We are coming up on two months, two long months of being in the hospital every single day. I feel like family and friends, and excellent medical care, have gotten Dylan this far but now, he needs even more support. I am exhausted and worn down. We have come to the limits of what we can do as a family, and the forty-five minutes of rehab three or four times per week from the hospital therapists, is just not enough. They are wonderful people, and they try very, very hard, but they have a full plate and Dylan needs more. Thumb wrestling and playing with a tennis ball have worked to this point. Dylan wasn't ready for more stimulation, but now he is. Dylan needs Craig Hospital.

Dylan is having a very sleepy day today. I guess that is best since hospital staff is very low due to the holiday. I don't know if there is such a thing as too much sleep for him right now. I will just sit here and pray today.

JULY 6, 2020 – FIFTY-FIVE DAYS SINCE THE ACCIDENT.

Burnout! This has already been such a long road, such a rollercoaster ride, and we are only eight weeks into it. I can now see why everyone was telling me to take care of myself. Physically is one thing, now that Matthew and Gabby can help, I only take eight-hour shifts. It feels so easy compared to the twelve-hour days. Mentally is an entirely different story. Much of the time now, Dylan refuses to do anything we try with him, which frustrates me. I want him working to get better. Dylan was a workout fiend in high school. He worked out more than I ever did, and when he saw the results, he was motivated to workout even more. I really want him out of a hospital setting and into a rehab. I want him to have access to and begin to build that workout mentality he used to have. I sure hope you can work the brain like other muscles. Don't get me wrong, I am very thankful to even be in this position. However, I need to keep further recovery for Dylan as my focus. This is our life now, and I am thankful for it.

JULY 10, 2020 – FIFTY-NINE DAYS SINCE THE ACCIDENT.

Dylan is sleeping a lot lately. He mostly sleeps all day, every day. I am not sure if that is OK or even normal for a TBI. No one at this hospital can really tell me either. He does seem to make strides when he is awake but mostly, I just sit in his room while he sleeps. He often sleeps through physical therapy or speech therapy when they do come see him. We are really at a point where we need a professional rehab. I believe they would be much better equipped to deal with him at this point.

Dylan was able to pass his swallow test and has been cleared to begin having pudding and ice cream. How great must that be for him to finally get food back in his mouth? Unfortunately, Dylan is not getting very excited over anything we bring him to eat. Is this all from the physical injury, or is he depressed? There is no way to know what he is thinking or feeling emotionally. How much does he remeber of his life before the accident? We could really use some experts to help us keep him motivated. Now and then, I give him a pep talk and he seems to respond for a little bit. I think if he is awake, he can understand. How do we get him to wake up more? This is a very long, slow road and every time we reach a milestone, there is another hurdle. Every time I think we are going to take off running toward recovery, there is a slowdown, or a setback. He has not said a word since those few words a few days ago. We are on a good path and ahead of where we were supposed to be, according to some doctors. I constantly remind myself that I am lucky and blessed to be here. Can anyone blame if I want more, and I want it now?

JULY 14, 2020 – SIXTY-THREE DAYS SINCE THE ACCIDENT.

I read a quote attributed to a Navy SEAL today that is perfect for me right now. "Most people fail out of SEAL training because they are waiting for it to end. Those who do well are usually only thinking about what is for breakfast." I am very focused on getting Dylan to Craig Hospital, and it is frustrating that it is taking so long. I need to focus on smaller things. I know the transfer is in the works. I need to think back to the hour-by-hour days. When he is awake, Dylan is doing amazing things. Yesterday he played Connect Four, tried to feed himself a little, and wrote a very sloppy "D" on a piece of paper. He didn't really **play** Connect Four, but when I handed him a chip, he would fight and fight to slowly move it to the drop slot and he seemed to understand that he was trying to get four in a row. Whenever he opens his eyes, I try to get him to do something, anything. I need to keep my focus on those moments and keep my attitude positive. I know this will all be a distant memory someday and I know my brain will likely filter out some of these bad memories. I thank God for getting me to this point.

JULY 15, 2020 – SIXTY-FOUR DAYS SINCE THE ACCIDENT.

Dylan continues to make some progress. Yesterday, with the help of PT, he was able to sit on the edge of the bed and hold his head up for five minutes. The therapist steadied him, and I held his tennis ball above my head for him to focus on. If he focuses on the tennis ball, he can hold his head up. It is hard to imagine, but these seemingly tiny movements are what he needs to start doing before we can get to the bigger movement. A few months ago, this kid could deadlift more than anyone on his football team, now it makes my day that he held his head up on his own for five straight minutes. Imagine what Craig Hospital will be able to do. There is a teleconference today between

Kaiser and Craig Hospital and hopefully an admission date will be set. I am hoping for next Wednesday, July 22, as the transfer date. Who gets to go along with him and when we get to visit with him is still to be decided. We have been talking about it and I think Gabby and Cindy are going to go with him, and I will relieve Cindy later. Our family comes together, and we always work out these issues with no problem. No one fights or bickers, and no one gets jealous or mad. We all share ideas and quickly come to the best solutions, no egos. It would be great if we can rotate our time with Dylan, but we will have to see what Craig Hospital's COVID visitation policy is by then. They have warned us that they take a conservative stance on trying to keep COVID out of their facility and that the policy can change at any time if new guidelines come out.

JULY 18, 2020 – SIXTY-SEVEN DAYS SINCE THE ACCIDENT.

Finally, a transfer plan. Dylan will be transferred to Craig Hospital on July 22. We have a call scheduled with Craig Hospital at nine a.m. on Monday morning to go over what exactly will occur. I know Dylan will be transferred via air ambulance. I cannot wait. I am super excited for him! Even if it means I will miss him terribly until I can get out there.

Dylan seems depressed to me. He doesn't want to do anything… ever! Right now, I have the TV on, and he seems to be watching it, but he will rarely even look at me. He eats and drinks very little. He has been in a hospital room for two months and six days. We all have. It is taking its toll. Craig Hospital should know how to handle this and how to get the most out of him. Before the accident, Dylan was so bright and full of life. It is very hard to see him like this, but it is much better than a few weeks ago. Stay positive and keep walking the road, this is another part of the journey.

JULY 21, 2020 – SEVENTY DAYS SINCE THE ACCIDENT.

Our time at Kaiser is finally coming to an end. Dylan has received great medical care here over the past forty-two days, including getting him a special mattress to help ward off bedsores. Now with the new hospital, the journey changes scenery. I am reflecting on these last seventy days. Ten weeks of sitting by his bed, alone. I have never been in Dylan's room with another family member there. There has not been a single day I have not been in the hospital, the same goes for Cindy. COVID has made this so much harder on us, but we have made it. Family and friends have supported us but could have helped so much more if they were allowed to. The support has been incredible. We got a few friends in to visit Dylan and lift his spirits, but that was shut down after just a few friends. The firemen and paramedics who first responded and are largely to be credited with saving Dylan's life, were able to get to see him briefly. Unfortunately, Dylan mostly slept through that visit and didn't get to thank them, but maybe one day.

Erica's time is mostly spent supporting me and handling everything back home. The kids, and other family members, all do what they can, and the community has been there for us the entire time. However, I am utterly exhausted and burnt out, but I can say I have made it this far. Dylan has also made it this far. I wonder what Dylan must be thinking. Does he have thoughts? I can't be sure what he recalls or even who he recognizes. He may know me one day and then not the next. I fight every day to stay positive and be happy with the progress he made. I can always bring him positive energy. He is going to the best place for him, and he has a chance. That's what all the praying has been for. I know he has more improvement in him, although admittedly, I wish I knew better what the result will be. Thankfully God has gotten him this far.

This morning, Dylan was sleeping when I first walked into the room. Within a few minutes, he opened his eyes and when I said good morning, he got a big smile on his face. What a wonderful thing to see…a smile. I bet if I ever read this journal back, a morning smile is exactly what I prayed for ten weeks ago. First, I prayed he would live, then I prayed he could be happy and smile. To get a smile is a true gift. I don't yet know how much I will get to see him at Craig Hospital. It might be a lot, or it may be seldom. I know that God is by his side either way.

With Dylan moving to Craig Hospital, I would enter a period where I spent less time at his bedside. I never thought about him any less, but I did journal less. I would journal during my time with him at Craig Hospital but if I was home, I only journaled if something major happened. Unfortunately, with this journey, too often the major things were negative.

Chapter **8**

ON TO CRAIG HOSPITAL

AUGUST 7, 2020 – EIGHTY-SEVEN DAYS SINCE THE ACCIDENT.

It has been a while since I journaled. Dylan was flown to Craig Hospital as planned on July 22. Cindy flew with him on the medical flight. She said he tolerated the flight well enough and carried his tennis ball with him. It was excruciatingly hard to not go with him myself. If it wasn't for COVID, I would have met him in Colorado right away. As it was, I had to wait two weeks. The first few days of that two weeks were unbearable. After being in the hospital with him and seeing him every day, I felt helpless, even more so than before. Suddenly I was not there, and I was at home trying to act as normal as possible. I tried to work as much as feasible but my ability to concentrate was low. I found it very difficult to sleep and often just laid in bed and cried. Having to go to the hospital and stay positive for Dylan had really helped me keep things together. I miss him so much. I need to be there with him. Eventually, the concentration part did get a little better over the two weeks. The missing him and getting emotional at night didn't really improve much.

A local restaurant reached out to us and wanted to help with a fundraiser. Dylan had introduced us to Kiki's Chicken Place and their legendary Kiki's Fries. The owners, Santiago and Summer Gonzalez, were having a grand opening for their newest location, close to Folsom High School, and they wanted to donate all of the proceeds from the day to Dylan's fund. As with other acts of kindness, this moved me to tears. Erica and I were not able to attend the grand opening because it happened to be the same day we were leaving to drive to Craig Hospital. I am not sure my emotions would have allowed me to attend anyway because from what I heard, the turnout was incredible. The lines were long all day, and everyone was talking about Dylan. The restaurant eventually ran out of certain items on their menu due to the overwhelming crowd. Erica's parents were able to attend and took Ty and Bella with them. When the Gonzalez family heard that Dylan's family was there, they refused to take any money for their meals. The outpouring of love was a tremendous spirit lifter and in the end, the Gonzalez family donated $10,000 to Dylan. What a beautiful gift from a super kind and loving family. Sadly, Summer Gonzalez would lose her battle with COVID a year and a half later.

Erica and I packed up Gabby's Jeep and left for Craig Hospital on Monday, August 3, 2020. Even Gabby's Jeep has a connection to this tragedy. I didn't get to go with her to pick it out. I didn't get to do the "dad thing" and help my daughter buy her first car. Pablo had to fill in for me while I was in the hospital with Dylan. So, driving it to Colorado with Erica is maybe a little therapeutic. We split the drive into two days and spent the first night in Salt Lake City. My only real memory of the night in Salt Lake City was walking down the streets of what felt like an abandoned city, unable to find a restaurant that was open for service, due to COVID. The next day we drove to Denver and spent a night at a hotel there before driving to Englewood, Colorado. This is where Craig Hospital is located. It wasn't a fun trip; it was a business trip. Our emotions were still raw, and we went through the motions to get there, but certainly didn't get to enjoy the trip. We met Gabby for lunch when we first got to Englewood and then went to Costco with her and stocked up on supplies for the apartment. The plan we have, is that we rented an apartment right down the street from Craig Hospital (they refer out to supply housing options, but at patient cost) and Gabby lives there full time. Due to COVID, Craig Hospital is only going to allow either me or Cindy to be with Dylan. Gabby stays in the apartment and prepares meals, does laundry, and is the shoulder to cry on when we get back each night. Gabby can work during the day, fulfilling her US Air Force ROTC duties and beginning her senior year of college. So, Cindy and I both take two-week shifts at a time because of the recurring airfare costs. We can get in to see Dylan starting each morning at eight a.m. and then we must leave at eight p.m. The twelve-hour days are long, and Dylan spends the night alone with the staff. Matthew wants to be a part of Dylan's care team, so he is coming out in a few days to give Gabby a little time off. Then he will return to California to complete his final year of law school. The amount of focus Gabby and Matthew have showed to be able to keep up at school AND to help with Dylan is incredible!

The schedule at Craig Hospital is intense. Dylan goes to therapies all day long and we go with him. Today for example, Dylan had an ear, nose, and throat checkup at 8:30 a.m. and then physical therapy from nine a.m. to ten a.m. In PT, the therapist strapped Dylan into a robot-looking machine to have him go through the motions of taking 1,000 steps. I was there and helped load him into, and out of, the machine. Craig Hospital encourages the caregivers, which is what I now am, to be very hands on. Everywhere we go there are electric lift systems built into the ceilings to help get the patients from their wheelchairs into a therapy machine, or into a bed. Dylan was awake and coherent enough to be able to push the button for the lift that lifts him out of his wheelchair and into the walking machine. It is incredible to see how this hospital is set up for the patients. After PT, I took Dylan to the exercise room and learned how to strap him into a peddling machine so that he could peddle for thirty minutes. We remove the foot pegs from Dylan's wheelchair and then lock the brakes, and set wedges against the wheels, so the chair stays stationary. Dylan's feet are then strapped onto the peddles. We start Dylan peddling and hope he peddles on his own, but if he stops peddling, the machine senses it and peddles for him. This way, Dylan's legs are still getting the movement. After thirty minutes the machine gives a readout letting you know how much work Dylan did by himself. Today, Dylan peddled for three miles and his muscle tension (which the machine also senses) went from a thirteen to a six. I am not exactly sure what everything means, but it all sounds way better than lying in a bed all day long. Dylan then had thirty minutes off before heading to speech therapy, where the therapist got him to shake his head no, eat some peaches, and play a bubble popping game on an iPad.

During the thirty-minute break, I tried to get Dylan to eat some Jell-O and he choked a little, scaring the heck out of me. When he was finished coughing, he said, "Damn it." That made us both laugh, it was the most beautiful little curse word I have ever heard. I got him to eat a little more before he quit. Dylan is being served pureed food and we sit beside him and feed him with a spoon. It might look kind of sad for people outside of the situation, but it is still progress for us. He doesn't eat enough to get all his calories, so he is also fed via feeding tube four times per day. I also told Dylan a story of another patient in the exercise room this morning. When the patient was being strapped into the bike, he yelled, "Ouch my balls." Dylan laughed at the story, so I know that silly little boy is still in there somewhere.

Today was a good day, but yesterday I was upset. It was my first day with Dylan and he was completely unresponsive. I even think his hands were not as relaxed as they had been back at Kaiser. The doctors here are trying different combinations of drugs to make him more alert. I was totally expecting to see big changes in Dylan after two weeks here, but my first day was kind of a bust. I know this is a journey and I know it will not be a straight line in recovery, but this road has proven to have twists and turns, and hills to climb that are beyond difficult. I was not ready for my first day to basically be watching him sleep. It was a bit of a punch in the gut, and I had to process it. Erica, my mom, and Gabby all talked to me and helped me organize my thoughts. I cried when I got back to the apartment with Gabby, but I got through it. Today was the reward, a day of accomplishments and progress. Thank you, God!

AUGUST 9, 2020 – EIGHTY-NINE DAYS SINCE THE ACCIDENT.

Today, we are on day four for me at Craig Hospital. My feeling at the beginning of this day four is that this is harder than I thought it would be. Gabby was able to have her first outside visit with Dylan today, and he was again 100 percent unresponsive, forgive about five minutes. Craig Hospital has a beautiful outside garden area, which I assume is usually used for large family visits. As part of their COVID plan, Craig Hospital is allowing limited, one-hour visits with one family member out in the garden area. The visit is supervised by a staff member to be sure we stay six feet apart and don't touch. I know there are reasons for these rules, but I am sure hugs would be therapeutic for Dylan right now. I tried everything I could think of to wake Dylan up—talking, touching, feeding, TV, arm wrestling—but nothing worked. It is very frustrating. Here he is, in the best hospital in the world for him, and he won't wake up. This is the place we fought to get him to, and he is sleeping through it. I needed to vent my frustration and get back to being positive. This is just how it goes. I have zero control over this, and I just need to keep walking the road. The doctors do not seem too worried. They know what they are doing and are doing their best.

I did get Dylan on the bike to peddle for thirty minutes again yesterday. His muscle tone went from a twenty-five to a five. About half of the time the machine was peddling for him and half the time he did it himself. If he can wake up, he can get better. I know it. Dylan is very left-leg dependent right now; his right leg is a weakness for him. He barely uses it. My job is to be here every day and take what I can get out of him, encourage him, and be his coach. On sleepy days, I just sit in his room and wait. I must keep in mind that those days are ok, and trust that God is still healing my boy. The good news about sleepy days is I can get my work done remotely.

Matthew comes to Colorado today and Gabby leaves. She has been a very big support system and my evening chats with her over a bottle of wine have really helped bring us closer. I am sure it will be the same with Matthew. We have another eleven a.m. outside visit scheduled with Gabby. The question is, "Will Dylan wake up to see her?" I will also make sure I get him on the bike again. Anything else we can accomplish will entirely depend on Dylan. One day…one hour at a time.

AUGUST 13, 2020 – NINETY-THREE DAYS SINCE THE ACCIDENT.

Every day is a gift. This is so true and today has been a better gift than usual. I feel like Dylan is really beginning to wake up. He has been much more alert this week, today especially. He is getting back some of the hand movements he was showing at Kaiser. Dylan lifted his leg today in physical therapy in a way I have not seen him do before. It is a small thing, but it makes me feel better to see even the smallest signs of progress. Keeping him awake for the day is always my biggest challenge. Today, speech therapy was helping Dylan learn to communicate using a clicker button. The therapist would play part of a video for Dylan and then pause it. Dylan had to click the clicker to get her to start the video again. The therapist asked me for a music video Dylan may like, and I thought of "Despacito" by Justin Bieber. I have the coolest memory of Dylan before the accident singing the entire song to me, word for word, in Spanish. He doesn't even speak Spanish, so it cracked me up. Dylan really seemed to respond to the video, and he participated in the session. When we got back to the room, Dylan and I shared a wonderful moment. Of course, I had the song in my head, so I sang just the word "Despacito" out loud, and Dylan looked at me and laughed. I know God is smiling on us today!

AUGUST 14, 2020 — NINETY-FOUR DAYS SINCE THE ACCIDENT.

It's Friday! Dylan has been sluggish this morning but that is probably because he had such an active week. The staff here warned me that this was likely to happen. Many patients tend to be exhausted by Friday because the week of therapies was so intense. Overall, I am now happy with the progress Dylan is making. He still has a long way to go, but I am excited to see him get some breakthroughs in physical movements. I believe once he gets motivated, his training ethic from football will kick in and he will make big gains. He currently likes to watch TV; it is probably what wakes him up the most.

SEPTEMBER 1, 2020 — ONE HUNDRED TWELVE DAYS SINCE THE ACCIDENT.

My first two-week shift with Dylan at Craig Hospital has ended and it was time to fly home to California. Erica had come to Colorado for the last few days so Gabby could spend some time with friends over the weekend. Gabby has wonderful, supportive friends who knew she could not get away, so they flew to Denver to cheer her up. The weather in Denver is crazy. It was near ninety degrees and beautiful when Erica got there, and when we were leaving on Tuesday, there was heavy snow. We were completely unprepared for the drastic change clothing-wise. The region went from summer weather to snow within thirty-six hours. Flying had always brought me a little anxiety and it was even more so for Erica. It was snowing heavily, and our plane was delayed right before takeoff to be deiced. This would normally unnerve me, and Erica would be near a full-blown panic attack. The recent tragedy had removed any fear of flying. I vividly recall looking at Erica and saying, "If this is how God wants us to go out now, I am fine with it." She readily agreed as we both leaned back and relaxed in our seats. An overwhelming sense of peace came over both of us.

I certainly would have liked to see more progress, but now I am hoping we will see a bump in recovery when Dylan gets his skull plates put back in. Currently Dylan is missing skull plates from both sides of his head and wears a protective helmet 24/7. There is nothing between Dylan's brain and the outside world except his skin. I could not imagine always living life with a helmet on, even to sleep. It seems so uncomfortable. The only time Dylan is without his helmet is when they take it off for five minutes to clean it. When his helmet is off, Dylan has big indents on both sides of his head. There is a piece of his skull about two inches wide, which runs down the middle of his head. The first time you see it, it makes your stomach sink. This is hard on all of us, but no one more than Dylan.

They eventually put Dylan's plates back in on August 26, 2020. He was about fourteen weeks without them overall. They used Dylan's original bone skull flaps, which had somehow trailed him to Colorado. I am not exactly sure how that worked. I know that Dylan's skull plates were frozen when they were first removed. They were kept at UC Davis Hospital for some time, and then eventually shipped to Colorado. There is debate in the medical community about whether it is better to use a patient's original skull plates, or whether it is better to go right to prosthetic skull plates. We were told the choice is ours, but how can we possibly know? Each surgeon has their own preference and the surgeon working on Dylan this time prefers to use Dylan's original bone skull plates, so that is what we went with. Dylan was transferred from Craig

Hospital to St. Joseph's Hospital, a Kaiser facility in Denver, for the surgery and stayed there while he recovered. Dylan was very swollen after the surgery and barely woke up for nearly a week. Cindy and Gabby went back to a twenty-four-hour bedside vigil while he was at St. Joseph's. They said the hospital was nice and they felt the surgeons did a good job, but a week back in the twenty-four-hour grind of a hospital was tough on them. Recovery is just so slow! Dylan is doing very little now, less than when I was there. When will we finally see some gains and keep them? How do I stay positive through this? Dylan now has a low-grade fever, so infection is a major concern. I cannot even imagine the setback he will suffer if he gets an infection. How much more of this can anyone take?

I fly to Denver tomorrow and will get to see Dylan on Thursday. The two-week rotation system we came up with seems to be working for us as Dylan's caretakers. Cindy and I switch every other Thursday. I will fly in on Wednesday evening. Cindy must leave Dylan's bedside at eight p.m. on Wednesday. I will head to the Hospital at eight a.m. on Thursday, and Cindy will fly home to California some time that same day. I am prepared for a little step back here as Dylan recovers. I just pray we see some improvements during my two weeks there. I fear we are coming to the end of in-patient rehab as far as what Kaiser will pay for. It is going to be scary and extremely expensive to get Dylan help when the insurance runs out. I remember when we were fighting to get Dylan to Craig Hospital, one of my coworkers asked me what I would do if we lost that battle. My answer then was that I will drain my work pension to pay for it if I must. I will do anything it takes to help my son. I remind myself to stop looking too far ahead. Worry can do nothing for me. Stay positive and stay in the now. As Erica says, "Close some of those open doors in your brain for now. They do not all need to be open at the same time." I am very tired!

SEPTEMBER 3, 2020 – ONE HUNDRED FOURTEEN DAYS SINCE THE ACCIDENT.

Did I mention this is difficult? I am with Dylan now. The surgery to replace Dylan's skull plates went well. He physically looks great with his head regaining its normal shape at last. Unfortunately, the surgery set him way back in his rehabilitation. There were some "c-acne bacteria" detected on Dylan's skull plates, so he is on antibiotics. C-acne bacteria, from what I understand, is a slow-growing type of bacteria that is often found on the skin's surface. But it can also be found many other places, especially following surgery. It degrades the skin and proteins that can in turn activate the immune system. Obviously, this can be a significant complication to someone in Dylan's condition because his immune system is already so compromised. He also has elevated heart rate and blood pressure, so he cannot go back on the stimulants, which were helping to wake him up. He is basically back to an unresponsive stage. He sleeps all day and does not respond to commands. He doesn't even open his eyes to watch TV.

I fight to try to stay positive. It feels so much like we are all the way back to square one. Will we ever see progress and then keep the progress? My positive thought for today is believing the progress will come now, since his skull plates are back in. We are heading into Labor Day weekend, so Dylan can take the next four days to rest. Hopefully after that, he can get back on his stimulants. The doctors tell me his brain is shaped properly and under the correct amount of pressure, so now my prayers are for there to be permanent gains and for them to come quickly. Cindy has a theory that part of Dylan's issue may have been something called "sunken brain syndrome," which basically means that because of Dylan's brain being misshapen for so long, it begins to have a deteriorating effect on cognitive function. We are learning all kinds of new things that we never wanted to know. I don't know if Cindy is correct, but no one seems to know. Please God, let us have some real recovery now. I really want to see Dylan make strides while he is here at Craig Hospital. As it stands now, the most alert Dylan has been since his accident was at Kaiser-Morse Hospital. But I do believe, and I do have faith. God has gotten us this far.

SEPTEMBER 6, 2020 – ONE HUNDRED SEVENTEEN DAYS SINCE THE ACCIDENT.

This journey is not for the faint of heart! They did tell us in the beginning that this was a long road with many peaks and valleys. Dylan's lead doctor at Craig Hospital warned us in the intake meeting that we need to consider this to be an eighteen-month to twenty-four-month injury at the very least. Remember when I said I would not make six months? You don't think you can, until you have no choice. If anyone had told me just how hard it would be to travel this road, I would never have believed I could make it. I have had hard times in my life but overall consider myself very lucky. With the adversities I have dealt with, I have always been able to have the inner confidence of being strong and pushing through. However, I was likely never really dealing with my deep-down true feelings. As it turns out, I was spoiled, and I didn't really appreciate it. Right now, I am not ok. I am not feeling strong, and I cannot lock these feelings inside. I play a dangerous game every day balancing positive vs. negative. If I give in to the negative, I get overwhelmed with a feeling that I can't do this. The truth is, right now Dylan is worse than when we brought him here. It was not supposed to be like that. We fought like mad to get him here. This is the place where miracles happen. We are at least halfway through our time here and his condition is inferior to when he arrived.

In another evil wrinkle to this, no one will say how long we can stay. Every two weeks they re-evaluate him until one day they will just say his "time's up." How is it that we are in the best hospital in the world for him and Dylan's condition is worsening? I can't think about that too long though. If I go down that rabbit hole, I am finished. Stay positive! His bone flaps are back in. He was awake when we came here. He will get back there once he heals a little. When he is awake, he can make progress. He is back to storming right now due to the surgery, so patience is the key. If the miracle must come after his time at Craig Hospital, then so be it. Negativity, even if rooted in the current reality, does me and more importantly, Dylan, no good. Keep fighting. Keep walking this road, this road we never chose to be on.

Chapter 9

FIGHTING THE INFECTION

SEPTEMBER 17, 2020 – ONE HUNDRED TWENTY-SEVEN DAYS SINCE THE ACCIDENT.

Today we received a brutal punch in the gut! I just spent a week at home expecting to come back to Dylan waking up and making great strides. Instead, I get a haymaker from my blind side. Dylan was diagnosed with an infection in his skull plates. Tuesday he was transferred back to St. Joseph's, and Wednesday he underwent four more hours of surgery to remove the infected plates and treat the infection. This was his fourth major surgery. A **HUGE** step backward. He will now undergo antibiotic treatment and wait six to eight weeks until he can have prosthetic skull plates put in. How much can this poor child endure? Why does it feel like he is being punished? I feel broken. I am taking this hard. I was mad, and sad, and inconsolable when I found out. Will he ever get better? It has been over four months since the accident. How long can we keep doing this? Have I just been kidding myself thinking he may ever get to a place where he can laugh and fish? Kaiser is bound to stop paying for his rehab soon. When that happens, we are going to have to do his rehab at home. This burden feels overwhelming.

I sit here now at Dylan's bedside in St. Joseph's Hospital while he lays in bed unresponsive. They say his surgery went well; I am thankful for that, but I have heard it before. They believe they found the small area of infection and attacked it. He is getting a new helmet made and will need to wear that helmet twenty-four hours per day for the next six to eight weeks. More steps backward. Dylan is currently in the ICU, but he will transfer out today. There is no way for me to know what even the near future holds. There is no sense in even trying to contemplate the things that will come. I will just continue to sit here and monitor his blood pressure and heart rate machines again and wait for ambiguous updates from the doctors and nurses, which end up leaving me more confused than anything. I will continue to pray he doesn't die. I will gladly take every little bit of progress I get when he finally does wake up. Now, my prayers include just getting him back to where he was when we came to Craig Hospital. What a cruel reality. I only have the strength to stay strong and positive because I want him to have that feeling in this room. I push all my anger and fear as far down inside me as I can, but this cannot be healthy. I pray, I look for positive signs, and I keep the hope. However, hope seems very far away right now. It's like a tiny speck of light that I can barely see. I just pray that light grows a little.

I now miss the walks to and from Craig Hospital. On my walk into Craig Hospital around 7:45 a.m., I would call my mom in Pennsylvania who was two hours ahead and talk with her about the day to come and do our best to keep each other positive. During the walk back to the apartment each night, I would call Erica who was one hour behind me and talk to her about how the day went and do our best to keep each other positive. I needed those conversations as emotional outlets. They gave me just enough strength to carry on. Here at St. Joseph's now, I sit by myself in the grim, cold corner, eerily like the early days of this tragedy and talk to only God. I can only pray He still has time to listen to me. I am stuck in my own pile of emotions; I am drained from the long journey already and fearful of what the road looks like ahead. No outlets, no reprieve, just the terrifying and draining feeling that I am in the same place I was months ago.

SEPTEMBER 20, 2020 — ONE HUNDRED THIRTY DAYS SINCE THE ACCIDENT.

This is unbelievable and pure torture! Dylan is back at Craig Hospital now, but he is completely unresponsive. I rarely see his eyes; they are always closed. Not only am I dealing with my unconscious and unresponsive son, but when the ambulance showed up at St. Joseph's to transport Dylan back to Craig Hospital, they told me they could not transport him unless I paid for the transport upfront, out of my own pocket. It was my insurance carrier, Kaiser Permanente, who called the ambulance. How can this be? Rather than trying to track down a live person at my insurance carrier and possibly cause a huge delay, I had to fish a credit card out of my wallet and pay for Dylan's transport. This is ridiculous!! Dylan made it back to Craig Hospital but that night I kind of lost it. I got very negative and let the haunting memory of Dr. Z's words creep into my mind. Maybe Dylan never wakes up. Why have we gone so far backward? Maybe I can't do this. How do I keep my sanity? What will happen to Dylan? I can no longer handle hearing people say, "It will be ok." It's not ok! It may never be ok! That is the reality.

On the way back to the apartment I stopped and bought a bottle of bourbon. Wine was not going to be strong enough tonight. I know I am drinking a little too much right now, but I need it to numb the pain and stop my brain at night. I got to the apartment where Gabby had made me dinner and had three big glasses of bourbon. I never do that! I vented and complained and cried to poor Gabby and then went to bed. I pray I am not making this even harder for her.

Today, despite being a little hungover, I have a better attitude. Dylan still did nothing all day, he is completely unresponsive, but I can accept this for now. I will just wait longer for the miracle. This whole journey is truly a journey of faith. If I lose faith, the journey will be over. It is not over yet. I assume the next few weeks will be spent trying to get Dylan to wake up. That's ok, I need to accept that and think of the steps that will inevitably follow. I need to have confidence that he will wake up someday soon.

SEPTEMBER 24, 2020 – ONE HUNDRED THIRTY-THREE DAYS SINCE THE ACCIDENT.

This entire experience is painfully lengthy and agonizing! Dylan is beginning to show signs of waking up, but it is very slow going. It is tough to get too excited when he does something he was doing months ago. Staying positive is a struggle. It is very important for me not to think too far down the road, however, at the same time, I need to think about how in the hell to get Dylan home. The staff at Craig Hospital are prepping Cindy and I to be his caregivers. They are teaching us the hands-on things we will need to do to care for Dylan by ourselves. Right now, Dylan eats through a feeding tube. He has strict times he takes certain medications that all look the same to me. He will need his mother and I to take turns to bathe him, as needed. He cannot use the bathroom by himself and wears a condom catheter twenty-four hours a day. There are so many little things that need to be done constantly just to care for him in the moment. Dylan cannot stand up, or turnover in bed. This is a lot. Are we really going to have to do all of this at home by ourselves? I guess it is like bringing a 220-lb. infant home from the hospital, which just so happens to be in another state. We will need a wheelchair van to get him home from the airport, yet we don't even have one. I feel so overwhelmed that my head is spinning.

I see other patients arrive at Craig Hospital in as bad of shape as Dylan, and then leaving a few months later in much better form than when they got here. There was a man from Southern California who was in a motorcycle accident, and his condition seemed similar to

Dylan's when we arrived. While I am shopping for a wheelchair van, his caregivers are learning how to help him transfer from a wheelchair into the front seat of a car, because he is finally awake and able to assist them. Why not Dylan? Another thing that this worldwide pandemic has robbed us of, is the ability to socialize with other caregivers at Craig Hospital. Being able to meet and speak with people going through the same things has been wonderful in the small doses we have gotten to. There is a cafeteria at Craig Hospital where normally the families would meet up and discuss the journey with their peers as they are going through it. We don't get any of that. We pass the other families in the hallway with masks over our faces. There is no connection with any other families or patients, which is making this journey even lonelier.

Why doesn't Dylan make the strides I see other patients make? Dylan just seems to get worse. Dylan just does not seem to respond to any rehabilitation whatsoever. Maybe we just need to take him home and work with him there. Perhaps it would behoove him to be out of the hospital setting. I am at least glad that the staff here has been so good at giving me a base of knowledge to be his caregiver. I am convinced the old Dylan is gone. My goal now is to make him happy and help him get to the point where he can experience joy. I don't know if that will be possible. We are at four and a half months since his accident and he still cannot do anything. He is not even back to swallowing pureed food again. He doesn't give a thumbs up like he used to. I just hold out hope that Dr. Z was wrong, and that God smiles on Dylan and helps him overcome this.

SEPTEMBER 26, 2020 — ONE HUNDRED THIRTY-SIX DAYS SINCE THE ACCIDENT.

Up, down, backward, and sideways, that is how this road goes. Dylan has had a reasonably good past few days. He is beginning to open his eyes more now. He is still not moving his hands or fingers, and still no thumbs up. He can barely squeeze my hand. Is he even squeezing, or I am just thinking he is squeezing? We just learned that Dylan's hemoglobin is at eight. A kid his age should be at fourteen. Low hemoglobin can cause fatigue and weakness. Given those symptoms, maybe I also have low hemoglobin! Dylan will now be getting iron IVs every day until his number comes up. I have high hopes that this will help wake him up. They are slowly increasing his stimulants again. However, my spirits are up for another reason as well. I told a Craig Hospital nurse that I was worried that Kaiser would force Dylan out of here soon and she said, "Oh, don't worry about that! This place has ways to keep patients here once we get them." I am taking that to heart. I want to stay right here and keep walking this road with Dylan. Keep walking forward with a slow and steady pace. I keep thanking God for the gains we have made and stay confident there will be many more to come.

SEPTEMBER 30, 2020 – ONE HUNDRED THIRTY-SEVEN DAYS SINCE THE ACCIDENT.

My two-week stint in Colorado this round is coming to an end. I will admit that it ended better than it began. Prayers are being answered, as Dylan is waking up a little bit. I now believe that we will not make huge strides until his prosthetic skull flaps go in, but he is opening his eyes and even laughed a few times. He still is not back to the Dylan we had before transferring to Craig Hospital, but there is hope. He is giving us signs that he can recover. When he is awake, he seems coherent. He seems to understand simple things and have emotions. I have hope again that he will now begin to progress. I know his physical strength still has a long way to go, but I am less worried about that because I know the strength he possesses physically. When we get him alert and awake, and normalize his brain pressures, hopefully that physical strength will quickly follow. The good news is that he is waking up and they have not yet reached the level of stimulants he was on before he had his skull plates removed again.

There is still room to go with these medications, or perhaps even different ones. Another beautiful thing about Craig Hospital is they are always trying new things. If one approach doesn't work, they find another. They use different types of drugs, different therapies, and they even switched Dylan's room so that he would get more direct sunlight to stimulate him awake. I know the sunlight helps me.

OCTOBER 17, 2020 – ONE HUNDRED FIFTY-FOUR DAYS SINCE THE ACCIDENT.

Frustration and patience; the rollercoaster continues. I am back in Colorado now. My life is strange. I probably cry more often when I am home because I have more time to reflect. I would say the truth is, things do not feel like they are going very well. Basically, Dylan is still not very alert, and he still doesn't do many of the things he did at Kaiser. He doesn't really use his hands at all. He will watch a movie or a video, and occasionally laugh. That is where I need to focus. He can laugh. I remember praying for that, I still pray for it. If we didn't have that right now, I would be crushed. To stay positive, I focus on that laugh. I pray and I hope that all the things he was doing and more will come back when he gets his prosthetic skull plates in. I will live with whatever God gives me, but caring for him at this level will admittedly be extremely difficult. By this weekend, we should be seeing the effect of a new stimulant drug they are trying, Bromocriptine. He just started taking it and I have seen no real difference yet. If I'm being honest, I really see no new changes in him from two weeks ago. We now have a little less than a month until his next surgery. The recovery from that surgery will have to be at a very rapid pace if we are going to get him anywhere close to where we wanted him to be when we leave Craig Hospital. Keep the faith, Paul! Keep walking the path! However, I am weary, and I get overwhelmed sometimes, but I promise I will never stop. Dylan will make it to the point where he can live a good life, he will be the one in a "Bagillion."

"Bagillion" is one of Dylan's nicknames. During his first year of football, when he was eight years old, Dylan was practicing on the offensive line with the scout team going against the first-team defense. The coach decided to make sure the defense was being honest and not jumping the snap, so he had the offense go on two. It worked and the defense jumped offsides. The defense got in trouble and may even have had to do up-downs, a famous football punishment tool. The scout team offense got back to the huddle, and they were all proud of themselves. Coach C asked the boys what they should do this time and Dylan spoke up and said, "Let's go on Bagillion." That's how the nickname was born.

Dylan was lucky enough to have the same core group of coaches for his first five or six years playing football. Most of them had sons on the team and eventually I joined in to help them. In every athlete's life there comes a time when it's probably better to have someone other than your parent coach you. When this time came and we no longer coached the boys, we all sat together in the stands to watch and help in other ways. One time when we were volunteering on the sideline for a freshman football game with all our boys playing, Dylan made a play from the defensive tackle position. He got in the backfield so quickly that he took the handoff from the QB before the running back got there. Dylan grabbed the ball and raced for a defensive touchdown. I remember Coach C there still referring to Dylan as "Bagillion" and saying, "That boy does something at least once every year to amaze me." We need those amazing things to happen now! C'mon, Bagillion!

OCTOBER 19, 2020 – ONE HUNDRED FIFTY-SIX DAYS SINCE THE ACCIDENT.

Now it feels like the torture just never stops. Yesterday and today, Dylan has been just **completely** unresponsive. We are all the way back to zero. When will the day come that he wakes up and stays awake? Again, I must keep my faith that getting the prosthetic skull flaps will be the key. We never really got to see what could happen with his skull back intact because the infection set in. Unfortunately, our time at Craig Hospital will not last long after the surgery. I wish there was a way to move the surgery up. I don't want another infection, but I so badly want those skull flaps back in. Please! I just need some steps forward without any steps back. I'm beginning to think that may be impossible.

OCTOBER 22, 2020 – ONE HUNDRED FIFTY-NINE DAYS SINCE THE ACCIDENT.

Oh, wow, the rollercoaster continues! After a terrible Sunday and Monday, Dylan is beginning to perk up again. Wednesday morning, he lifted his left thumb up and down on command. He has not done that in weeks. On Thursday morning, he had a great occupational therapy where he held his head up on his own for long stretches of time. This is true emotional confusion. One minute I want to scream, and the next minute I am overcome with joy. I try to keep my eyes up and my head forward, but doubts and fears are everywhere, and time seems to be their ally. I believe that once Dylan's brain is shaped normally again and once his brain pressure equalizes, we will be able to make the gains we are seeking. In the beginning, I was praying that Dylan would not need a permanent shunt in his brain, but now I really don't care. I see other patients here making great strides and yet Dylan has not. If a shunt means a better life, then I am all for it. The doctors have no idea if he will need one yet. In this instance, I find myself jumping ahead.

OCTOBER 26, 2020 – ONE HUNDRED SIXTY-THREE DAYS SINCE THE ACCIDENT.

Everyone gets better except for Dylan! Patients I have seen here since Dylan arrived are on the mend. These patients wake up, they improve…not my son. They walk, sometimes practicing their steps in the hallway in front of Dylan's room. They talk…their loved ones get the chance to hear their voices again…but not Dylan…not me. I am happy for them, but I am very worried for Dylan. I guess I need to be prepared to take him home like this and care for him as best I can. Maybe his injuries are just as bad as Dr. Z said and there is nothing that can be done…will we never see those advances?

I now feel like we are 100 percent wasting our time at Craig Hospital. Dylan is getting nothing out of the therapies they try to provide. I must hand it to the therapists because despite the repeated failures, they still try several times each day to get Dylan to respond. It is a shame that the American health care system with insurance is so complicated and often backward that they could not just have transferred Dylan to a care facility when he was diagnosed with the infection. They could have paused the clock on the rehab. Dylan is an eighteen-year-old boy/man with a long life ahead of him, but a few dollars to an insurance company determines what may be lifelong consequences for him. Maybe if they paused his rehab, Dylan could get his prosthetic plates and begin to wake up. Then he could be transferred back to Craig Hospital and be able to participate in his rehabilitation. Being at Craig Hospital right now and wheeling Dylan around to his different therapies feels like a complete waste of time. This is so frustrating. Maybe Cindy is correct, and Dylan has sunken brain syndrome. I believe we may be at a point where we need to consider moving the surgery up. It may mean a little more risk of another infection, but we must get him more responsive.

OCTOBER 27, 2020 – ONE HUNDRED SIXTY-FOUR DAYS SINCE THE ACCIDENT.

Today was another tough day. Dylan has been unresponsive all day again. I have made sure the Craig doctors know Dylan has been unresponsive for days. Perhaps they will consider moving up his surgery. I don't know what they will decide, but I want them to consider all options.

On a different, but related front, I have heard that Kaiser is refusing to extend Dylan's time at Craig Hospital past November 5. Dylan's surgery will likely be on November 11, so I believe they will extend his timeline some, but any real recovery at Craig Hospital seems unlikely now. I have sent a message to the Kaiser ombudsman again to try to begin a dialogue. We are absolutely prepared to fight like hell to get Dylan's stay extended here. I know that insurance companies just count the weeks that someone is in a rehab, but Dylan has been sick most of his time here. He is an eighteen-year-old boy, he deserves to receive every opportunity available to him to help his recovery. His life is worth at least that! I know the Craig Hospital doctors are fighting to keep Dylan and I will probably never fully know all they have done to keep him this long. How can Kaiser quit on him? Is that what's happening? Or is this helpless feeling I am having spilling over into everything I'm thinking? I feel like all my hopes now ride on Dylan's rebounding after this next surgery. All this time at Craig Hospital feels worthless as far as his recovery goes. The real value to our stay here is that they have forced Dylan to move and have stimulated his muscles so there is less atrophy. The other positive is that I now know how to use all the equipment I will need to take care of him at home. That alone is priceless. I can feel that this recovery burden is switching to the shoulders of the family. We will not have all the fancy equipment they have at Craig Hospital, but we will battle like mad to keep Dylan's recovery going.

OCTOBER 28, 2020 – ONE HUNDRED SIXTY-FIVE DAYS SINCE THE ACCIDENT.

Today is my last day with Dylan for a while. God has sure made me stronger. I feel bad when my weaknesses show up and my family sees it or senses it, but I need to get it out sometimes. I can feel that something is not right with Dylan. I know not having his skull flaps in is setting him back. He needs to have this surgery to begin moving forward again. He goes for a CAT scan tomorrow and if it shows sunken brain syndrome, he may go into his surgery sooner than currently planned. That worries me due to the infection risks but excites me because I want him to get better. Today, Dylan's main doctor told me that he is concerned that Kaiser may transfer Dylan to St. Joseph's for the surgery and then not allow him back to Craig Hospital. That both worries and infuriates me. I called and spoke with the ombudsman from Kaiser again and she at least seemed to listen to me. She at least pretended to have empathy. She informed me that she will get back to me in a few days. I made sure she knew that if Kaiser did something sneaky like that, Dylan's entire family and the giant community following and praying for him would be irate. Hopefully that works, but just in case, Matthew is talking with one of his professors about what it would take to appeal any decision Kaiser makes to send Dylan home.

NOVEMBER 12, 2020 – ONE HUNDRED EIGHTY DAYS SINCE THE ACCIDENT.

This morning there is yet another delay! I was supposed to be at St. Joseph's Hospital right now, but they delayed Dylan's surgery. This was a Kaiser decision; I am told due to operating room availability. COVID has all hospitals in the country under stress. Cindy's two weeks with Dylan were a little better as he woke up a little bit for her. They stopped giving him Bromocriptine and put him back on Amantadine and that seems to have helped some. It's not much, but at least he is awake a little bit. Our time here at Craig Hospital is coming to its conclusion. Recovery wise, it has been a giant disappointment, but it is what it is. This is part of my journey. It just wasn't meant for Dylan to get better here. If he is ever going to have improvement, now it will be at home with his family and friends.

Today is six months since the accident. I have done a decent job lately of burying the "what if" feelings. Things like: What would life be like right now if Dylan didn't get hurt? Would he be playing football for Moravian University? Would he have a career in the medical field? Would he desire to have a future family? However, I concentrate more now on how to give him a quality of life, and how to give him some happiness. I realize that I will likely be caring for him for the rest of my life. I just need him to get back some of his gains; to smile and laugh and communicate. If he can just get control of his bathroom stuff and eat real food again, that would be a major win.

Erica and I had an interesting and sobering conversation last night. She is worried that I am burying my grief for what Dylan's life "could have been." That perhaps, I'm not being honest with myself. If I wasn't, would I even be aware of it? She assured me that it is ok to have those feelings and that they are valid and real. She wanted to emphasize it would be appropriate for me to acknowledge them and it was ok to mourn "what could have been"…and then we move on…together. For now, I will just keep praying and keep walking the road.

NOVEMBER 13, 2020 – ONE HUNDRED EIGHT-ONE DAYS SINCE THE ACCIDENT.

We just finished a speech therapy session outside in the garden. Donna is in town giving Gabby a little time away. The amount of support that Gabby and Matthew have been giving is truly incredible. I know so many members in my family wish they could help us more, but with COVID, that is just not possible. The outdoor speech therapy was a brutal session. I had to physically hold Dylan's eyes open so that he could participate. On a good note, Dylan did participate when I held his eyes open. The speech therapist would hold up two NFL team logos and would ask Dylan to stare at the one which will win this week. She did the same thing last week, and the therapist said Dylan was rather successful in her family betting pool. Again, a small slice of normal.

It does give me some hope that if we can wake Dylan up, he is in there. If the skull flaps help him to wake up, I believe he can make huge improvements. This is where my hope lies now. Why be anything but positive? I no longer want to speak with anyone about what Dylan's life could have been or should have been. There is only what is. This is his path, and this is my path. Why look at it any other way? I have hope. If the skull flaps don't immediately result in great improvement, I will still have hope. I will always keep hope for the smallest of improvements. Anything to make Dylan's life a little better.

Chapter 10

IT IS NEVER EASY

NOVEMBER 15, 2020 – ONE HUNDRED EIGHTY-THREE DAYS SINCE THE ACCIDENT.

Here we go! Tomorrow morning Dylan will be transported to St. Joseph's Hospital. Surgery will be on Tuesday morning. Today, Dylan slept all day, including through an outside visit with Donna. I so wish he could wake up and see all the support from those who love him. Donna flew to Colorado to give Gabby a much-needed break and take over the duties in the apartment, but she also wanted to see Dylan. Maybe she could do something to try to help stimulate him. After the visit with Donna around 4:30 p.m., I noticed Dylan's eyes were open. He looked at me and seemed alert. I began to explain to him what his week held, the hospital transfer, the surgery. He seemed to get sad. I think he is aware enough to dread the surgery. I explained to him that Gabby and I will be with him twenty-four hours a day, and that he will feel much better once it is finished. If he has headaches or feels sick now, this will make that stop. This is now his fifth surgery in six months and with any luck, the last one. I hold out hope that the road will all be about recovery now. When I finished speaking with him, he seemed better, so and I said, "If you understand me, blink twice," and he did! **Two perfect, slow, deliberate blinks.** I know that was God making him coherent enough to get that bit of communication with me. I feel better now, and I cannot wait for healing.

Lately it has been a little tough talking about Dylan's progress with family and friends. I must go over everything two or three times as I update everyone. I went through everything again with Donna last night. It is hard because I feel like every time I tell the story, I am reliving it. I know I can get through this, but the reliving it repeatedly is tough. I guess it must come out though, I can't just keep it inside. I've been told that sometimes, in the retelling of his accident, it can help reduce its impact on my soul. That I heal a little more each time, with every moment I relive the pain. I don't know about all that, but as it turns out, I'm getting practice at it…whether I want to, or not.

NOVEMBER 18, 2020 — ONE HUNDRED EIGHTY-SIX DAYS SINCE THE ACCIDENT.

I wanted this to be a happier entry, but this journey can just never be easy. The surgery went well yesterday, but soon after it ended, Dylan suffered some small seizures. I was not there for the seizures but walked into the room just after they stopped. I immediately noticed he was breathing funny. They took him for a CT scan, the second one in less than an hour, and saw no changes in his brain. That is the good news. Gabby took the overnight shift and the next morning said they detected another small seizure. They decided to heavily sedate him and put a breathing tube back in him. He had some more small seizure activity overnight and they say his pupils seem less reactive now. Dylan received another CT in the morning and, thankfully, they again saw no changes in the brain. I spoke with Dr. R this morning, and he believes Dylan may be having one long seizure, which has never ended. He equated it to a computer freezing and you get that little spinning wheel. He believes Dylan's brain may have expanded back to its normal shape more quickly than anticipated, and that caused it to sort of short circuit a bit. There is no way to know how long the seizure activity will last. Dylan now has an EEG hooked up to his head and they are monitoring his brain activity remotely and constantly. They have increased his anti-seizure meds and now we just wait. Dr. R said to "buckle up" because there is no telling how long we will be in this stage. This journey is truly pushing me to the edge. Every time I think I cannot handle any more, something more occurs. What ever happened to "God never gives you more than you can handle"? I am pretty certain I am near my end.

NOVEMBER 20, 2020 – ONE HUNDRED EIGHTY-EIGHT DAYS SINCE THE ACCIDENT.

Just when I believe we are getting somewhere, we end up losing more ground. Yesterday morning St. Joseph's Hospital went into COVID emergency protocol and transferred all ICU patients into what used to be the Neonatal Intensive Care Unit. Dylan, who previously had a private room with the lights low, temperature down and visitation to a minimum, now must share a room with another ICU patient and the staff seems to be figuring everything out on the fly. It feels more like a temporary hospital set up in a natural disaster. Dylan needs peace and quiet and this is the exact opposite. All the nurses are confused as to where anything is, where things go, and what the current visitation rules are. Not to mention they all are clearly overworked. I had another small breakdown today and yelled at someone who would not let me through the doors to get to Dylan's room. I feel like the entire world is tense right now and everything becomes a struggle for me. I know I am not myself right now, I don't have any patience to deal with people.

The wife of Dylan's new roommate is speaking on speaker phone giving updates to her family on their loved one's condition. Normally that would be a wonderful thing, but Dylan is supposed to have no stimulation and peace and quiet as he recovers from the surgery and tries to stop having seizures. Instead, this already small room has been divided in two, via a curtain. The room is so crammed that at one point, I had to slide my chair into the hallway so the hospital staff could wheel an X-ray machine into Dylan's roommate. This road has been hell already and now this. I silently sit here while there are bright lights and loud noises around my gravely injured son, who is not to be stimulated. It is torture, on top of torture. This COVID is such a confusing medical-political topic. I have not had the time or energy to really focus on what is true and what is outright lies about the virus for the past six months. With all the different medical facilities Dylan has been admitted to, we constantly must trust new medical staff with our son's life. Craig Hospital understands the special needs of a TBI patient, but in the ICU, Dylan is just another patient. The staff needs to understand the negative effect the COVID restrictions are having on Dylan, and I am the only one here who can fight for him. These effects could possibly last the rest of his life, not just the moment. I just pray that these COVID emergency protocols are necessary, or I hope the people overacting to this situation get what is coming to them.

Because of this COVID emergency, Gabby could only stay with Dylan until eleven p.m. and I was allowed to come back to see him at seven a.m. Again, new rules to adjust to. When Gabby left at eleven p.m., Dylan was down to 5 mg of Propofol an hour and the plan was to remove the breathing tube in the morning. I walked into Dylan's room at seven a.m. and the nurse told me that after eleven p.m. last night, a call came in from the neurologist watching the EEG remotely saying that Dylan had a two-minute seizure around 7:30 p.m. last night. This means Gabby was there but neither her, nor the nurses were able to detect it. Because of the seizure, they increased the propofol to 20 mg and started a Versed drip. They will re-evaluate Dylan this morning. This honestly may kill me; I am losing hope.

NOVEMBER 21, 2020 – ONE HUNDRED EIGHTY-NINE DAYS SINCE THE ACCIDENT.

It turns out that Dylan also had a seizure at nine p.m. that night, but none since. It has now been close to forty-eight hours with no seizures. They removed the Propofol medicine sometime overnight. Now they are reducing the Versed from six to zero over the next twenty-four hours. They will now introduce anti-seizure meds into Dylan's treatment plan and see what works best. I don't know what will happen when he goes on anti-seizure meds. I hear they can make people sleepy and that is the last thing Dylan needs. Dylan has still not opened his eyes since the surgery. Hopefully, he can begin to wake up soon. I really want that breathing tube to come out. They told me he needs to be awake to get it out. He has never had trouble breathing and I am sure that tube is uncomfortable for him.

This room sharing due to the COVID emergency has not gone smoothly. Dylan is sharing a room with Randy, an older gentleman on his fourth brain surgery. Dylan is supposed to be in a low-stimulation environment, but instead there is always a lot going on in his room. Dana, Randy's wife, naturally must update family members on how he is doing. That is not her fault, but it creates noises Dylan normally would not have to deal with. I have complained to every nurse and doctor who comes in, and anyone else who will listen. Please find my son a room in this hospital, a broom closet if you must, where he can have low stimulation!

Then things went from bad to worse. Around four p.m., Randy started having trouble breathing and the nurse had to call a "code blue." Within minutes, there were seemingly thirty people in and around Dylan's room. Dana and I were herded into the hallway and could only watch through the window as the staff filled the room and worked on Randy. I could barely see Dylan due to all the people around him. This is the exact opposite of low stimulation. I'm extremely thankful they were able to get Randy breathing again. I certainly don't want to see anyone die. This stimulation is exactly what Dylan does **not** need. My reoccurring, constant thoughts are that he needs quiet, this is terrible. After the code blue, I again spoke with the charge nurse about getting Dylan a low-stimulation room. She had a little bit of an attitude in the beginning because she thought I was just demanding a private room. I understand this COVID emergency protocol situation is high stress for everyone, especially nurses. My mom and sister are nurses, I understand it is a tough job. However, I have one job here and it is to help Dylan. I speak when he cannot speak. I will not fail at my job.

As I spoke with the charge nurse, I got emotional, kind of like when I confronted the patient advocate about her flippant answer to getting Dylan into Craig Hospital. Tears were streaming down my cheeks as I explained to her that Dylan is a TBI patient who is suffering from seizures. His brain needs to rest and heal. All this stimulation is not good for him, in fact, I have been told it is very bad for him. I saw her eyes begin to well up with tears also. I know the pressure on this medical staff in this COVID emergency was unfathomable. They were all overworked and probably worried about their own health and safety, not to mention their loved ones. She began to try to think of options with me, but ultimately there were none. All I could do was go back to my chair and pray. Now I can pray for Dylan **and** Randy. Randy was heavily sedated now, so the next few hours were very quiet. The charge nurse later came to check on Dylan and explained that she understood that I was only trying to look out for Dylan. I am glad she recognized it, but really, she had no idea how long I had been fighting this battle.

When all had quieted down, I snuck out to the bathroom and made a quick call to Erica. I was able to text her during the code blue, but this was the first time I had talked to her. I was obviously upset, and my emotion was coming out as anger. Erica said to me, "Sometimes God puts people in our lives for a reason. Try to find the reason Randy and Dana have been put there." Later that the day, I got to have a conversation with Dana while both our loved ones slept with breathing tubes down their throats. Dana is an exceptionally warm and kind person and she listened to Dylan's story and was moved by it. She offered her best wishes and even offered me a little bag of snacks she had with her. It turns out Randy had done some work installing automatic doors at Craig Hospital, so they understood what Dylan was going through…at least a little bit.

NOVEMBER 22, 2020 – ONE HUNDRED NINETY DAYS SINCE THE ACCIDENT.

Oh, boy, where do I begin? The next day, I saw Dana in the lobby and she handed me a Dick's Sporting Goods bag. She had gone out and bought Dylan a Denver Broncos shirt for when he wakes up. What a beautiful gesture, for her to stop and do something so nice for a stranger, when her own loved one is going through a tough time. It is just incredible. Again, this is renewing my faith in humanity. Randy had surgery and was stable now. He has a tracheotomy in, so no more breathing issues. Dana thinks that is best for him. As it turns out, God did put Randy and Dana in my life for a reason and maybe it was to remind me how wonderful people can be.

Dylan got his breathing tube out and was moved to an intermediate care unit, ironically a single room. He has not really rebounded like I had hoped but he is opening his eyes a little. I noticed Dylan's heart rate was strangely low while he slept, like in the sixties and seventies. I think this is a good sign since I have not seen it that low. Unfortunately, twenty-four hours later it was back to the nineties, where it has been most often throughout the injury. However, I'm not sure what it means, I was hoping it meant his brain had kind of normalized and he was in a deep, relaxing sleep. Dylan was awake for maybe an hour today. His eyes opened but he had no real interaction. He seemed to watch TV some of the time. I don't know what to think any more. I just sit here and say my prayers. The feelings of sadness and isolation have become excruciating at this point. I cry. I pray. I gain hope. I lose it. This feels like a cruel nightmare that won't end. I'm still terrified that even when it eventually does, it won't end the way I'm praying. This lack of control is enough for my anxiety to bore its way through the small dose of medication I take to keep it at bay.

The infectious disease doctor came in and told me some bacteria had grown in the cultures taken during Dylan's surgery. To summarize, we can never win. Dylan will need to be on two antibiotics for the next six weeks, so he will need to have a PICC (Peripherally Inserted Central Catheter) line in his arm. Dylan may need to be on Doxycycline for the rest of his life, but I don't really care about that right now. I now focus my prayers on keeping the infection away; Dylan needs a break. I hope infection is not the reason for his heart rate increase. I sit here and I worry. I feel deflated sometimes and then remember not to waste my energy on those feelings. Think positive thoughts, bring positive energy to Dylan. Every time Dylan opens his eyes, I tell him everything will be ok now. He will be getting better, and aesthetically, he looks much better with his skull plates back. I fight back the negative, but it's a struggle to say the least. I overemphasize the positive. When I can distract myself, I do. I am on leave this week from work, but I find myself working anyway because it is a good escape.

NOVEMBER 25, 2020 – ONE HUNDRED NINETY-THREE DAYS SINCE THE ACCIDENT.

It has been a positive twenty-four hours. Gabby relieved me at seven p.m. last night and said Dylan woke up and watched a movie with her until one a.m. Knowing that, I expected today to be another sleepy day, but Dylan woke up at eight a.m. and watched movies with me until almost noon. I did a little eye tracking therapy with him. He watched short videos on my phone, and I moved it around, so he had to follow. He did well, not great, but it was something. He is still not moving his hands at all but hopefully will soon.

Craig Hospital said they are setting up a transport to get Dylan back there today at one p.m. They said they will bend the rules and accept him back even if his COVID test results are not back yet. Every time Dylan transfers hospitals, he must have a negative COVID test right before leaving. If the results are not back, Craig Hospital is willing to isolate him until we get the negative test. If by chance he was COVID positive, they would have to transfer him back to St. Joseph's. I am going to try my best to not let my thoughts even go there, but I admit, it was a fight to keep the worry out of my mind. I woke up this morning at 3:30 a.m. and laid in bed obsessing about that stupid test. I never did go back to sleep. Worry and doubt about things I have no control over is maybe the hardest part of this journey for me.

Kaiser ultimately agreed to give Dylan two weeks at Craig Hospital after his return. Cindy was covering those two weeks, and while we heard Dylan was making a little progress, it was minimal. Two weeks? He was recovering from his fifth major surgery. A surgery he needed because he got an infection during a surgery at a Kaiser hospital! Two weeks? We were told you don't get a second chance at in-patient rehab, so this is Dylan's last two weeks in the place where miracles happen. It was a tough pill to swallow.

When the time came, Pablo flew to Colorado to help Cindy deal with Dylan on the flight home. Typically, Craig Hospital would send a nurse along on the flight and have her stay a few days to help get Dylan settled, but due to COVID, that was not allowed. Dylan is semi-conscious at best. He had to be loaded onto a commercial flight using a special wheelchair that fit down the aisle. He was then strapped into the middle seat using the seat belt and a second strap placed around his chest to keep him leaning back in his seat. He had a feeding tube in his stomach and a condom catheter on. Cindy and Pablo managed to make it, but this was supposed to be a triumphant return from Craig Hospital, and clearly it wasn't.

Dylan needed a wheelchair van to get him home from the airport. We had not had time to buy one, so we posted on social media that we needed to borrow one. In another beautiful sign of the community love we have experienced, a girl who had gone to school with Dylan found out about our request. She asked her dad to help. Her dad was the manager of a specialty shop in Sacramento that sold wheelchair vans, of all things. He reached out to us and offered us a free one-day rental to get Dylan home. Erica and I picked up the van and met Pablo, Cindy, and Dylan at the airport. We managed to get Dylan into Cindy's house where we had bought wheelchair ramps and had rented medical equipment delivered.

Chapter 11

THE HIDDEN MONSTER

Dylan has been home for two weeks and it is HARD! His first afternoon at home was nice, as we all sat around at Cindy's house and told Dylan stories. He moved his head and his eyes and tracked us all as we spoke. He seemed to like being home. He is at Cindy's house full time right now because we only have equipment for one household. It is impossible to transfer his stuff from house to house, as it is extensive and just not practical. This seems tough on Cindy. Dylan requires full twenty-four-hour, around-the-clock care. Dylan cannot hold his head up very well on his own, so he has a special head rest attached to his wheelchair. He cannot control his saliva, so we keep a drool cloth on his chest, and we must wipe his mouth often.

We are all extremely busy trying to organize a routine to care for him. Poor Erica, I drag her along gathering items we need to set up our house from people selling the equipment on Craigslist. The caretaker task must be shared. It is too much for one person. So, to have Dylan at our home as well, we need things like a hospital bed and Hoyer lift. We hope to share Dylan between Cindy's house and our house on a weekly basis. Insurance covered **one** of every item, but we need two. We are buying what we need using the money people have donated. Caring for Dylan is so intense that we need a week of rest after having him for a week. I found a hospital bed and Hoyer lift on Craigslist from a nice couple in Rancho Cordova, California. We shared Dylan's story as we were picking up the items and they were so moved that they threw in some additional care items they could spare.

We had the carpet removed from the downstairs bedroom in our rental house and had vinyl flooring installed. Our friend Terrance, whose son Lucas was with Dylan the night of the accident, paid for the install. I joined a Facebook group for wheelchair vans and found one we could afford. Unfortunately, Erica, Bella, and I had to fly to Las Vegas, rent a car, and then drive to Lake Havasu, Arizona, to purchase it. We stayed the night with a cousin of Erica's and drove the van home over the next couple of days. Gathering what we need is exhausting and we have not even had Dylan overnight at our house yet. The struggle is real.

The community wanted to show their support for Dylan, and again, because of COVID, having everyone over was not an option. They came up with the idea of having a small parade of cars loaded with Dylan's friends and family drive by Cindy's house and honk and wave. All we had to do was sit with Dylan at the end of Cindy's driveway. It was a beautiful gesture and I thought it was a good idea at the time, but it didn't work out that way. Dylan was wholly unresponsive the day of the parade. He sat in his wheelchair with his drool bib and a special strap attachment to hold his head upright. We had been keeping people posted about his condition, but I am sure seeing him was hard to swallow. I know it was for us. Erica and Gabby even tried holding Dylan's eyes open like we sometimes did at Craig Hospital to see if it would stir Dylan awake. Car after car drove by, honking and waving, some even crying. Others made posters. We also had balloons to show Dylan that this was a celebration. This scene was hard on me. It really bothered me to be showing Dylan this way. I had it in my head that this was going to be a heroic parade celebrating Dylan's recovery, but instead, he was comatose. I had a bit of a mental breakdown. I felt sick to my stomach and just wanted the parade over. I got my hands on some bourbon and had a few shots to numb the anguish. By the time it was over, Erica had to drive me home. The only consoling factor is that everyone seems to truly understand and empathize with our pain. It seems strange that they could, but somehow, they do.

On Christmas Eve, for the first time since May 11, 2020, Dylan came to our house. It was just a visit, but he was here for a few hours to celebrate. It was very emotional to have him here. Nani and Papi (Erica's parents) came over. My favorite part was when we FaceTimed my mom and Dylan blinked one time to confirm that he wanted her to buy him some new Van's sneakers for Christmas. It really felt like he understood the question. Little things like this keep my hopes alive that as he weens off the anti-seizure meds, he will recover even further. The doctors have outlined a six-month plan to get Dylan off the anti-seizure meds and back on stimulants. Dylan's six-week course of antibiotics ends tomorrow. He has an EEG to check for seizure activity next Tuesday and then it is all up to us. Now that we have him home, let's walk this path slow and steady, please God.

The Fritz family gave us a standing chair. This is a special chair which once we transfer Dylan into the chair from his wheelchair, we can pump him up to a standing position. This is far below the level of machines they used at Craig Hospital, but it does work some of his muscles and Dylan has been doing well with it. We were forced out of a hospital with literally millions of dollars' worth of equipment to rehab Dylan, into our home with a second-hand portable Hoyer lift and a donated standing chair. It doesn't feel like it should be this way, but we will keep going. I am both excited and nervous for Dylan to come spend his first full week at our house.

DECEMBER 31, 2020 – TWO HUNDRED THIRTY DAYS SINCE THE ACCIDENT.

Just when you think it can't get any shittier, things get shittier! On Tuesday night I got a call from Gabby that Dylan needed to go to the emergency room. Dylan was at Cindy's house, but I had the wheelchair van at my house, because Cindy lives in a community where parking is difficult. I drove the ten-minute drive to get him. Dylan had the EEG earlier in the day at Kaiser Medical Offices in Roseville, California. Gabby had driven him there in the van. Dylan threw up soon after they arrived at the appointment, but everyone assumed he was probably car sick. They were still able to do the EEG. Dylan was ok for the ride home but threw up again at dinner time. Cindy called the Kaiser advice line to ask what to do and was told to take him to the Kaiser emergency room in Roseville for evaluation.

When I got to Cindy's house, Gabby and I loaded Dylan into the van. At that time, I will admit I thought it was overreacting a little to take him to the ER for two vomits, but I went with it. Roseville is about a forty-five-minute drive from Cindy's house. Gabby and I only made it about a mile and a half from Cindy's house when Dylan vomited again, this time all over himself and the inside of the van. As a parent, I have dealt with kids vomiting in the car before. Dylan was not able to help direct where he vomited. I pulled to the side of the road and climbed into the back to make sure Dylan was still breathing and clean the vomit off him. The van was the type which had a ramp that we use to wheel Dylan into the van and then he was able to stay in his wheelchair, and we strapped the chair down to the floor of the van with special tie downs for safe transport.

I made the decision to have Gabby call Cindy and instruct her to dial 911 and have an ambulance meet us at her house. It was just too hard to control Dylan and we had too far to go to get to the ER. I knelt on the floor of the van and held a vomit bag at Dylan's mouth while Gabby drove the van back to Cindy's. EMS arrived at Cindy's at the same time we did. That's the second time they were there with an incredible response time. We got Dylan out of the van and into the driveway so they could begin to assess him. Some of the crew was gathering info from us, while others took Dylan's vitals. They initially agreed to transport Dylan to Kaiser-Roseville ER, but that was before they saw his vital signs. Dylan's blood pressure was so low and heart rate so high that their protocols dictated that Dylan had to go to the closest hospital. This meant Dylan had to be taken to Mercy Hospital in Folsom. A lower-level trauma emergency room, but the closest drive time. I was in shock that this had become such a dire emergency. I just thought he was vomiting.

The ambulance left with Dylan and I drove the van to Mercy Hospital; I would need it to bring Dylan home, I would hope. Of course, these are COVID times, so nothing can be easy. They would not let me in the ER. Apparently, Mercy Hospital-Folsom's COVID rules were to admit the patient and isolate him until he tested negative for COVID. Once Dylan tested negative, they would let me in to be by his side. I still didn't understand what was going on. They sent me home to wait until Dylan passed his COVID test. I can't really say I was upset. I think I was more in shock, dazed, and confused. Luckily, I was only home about an hour when they called me to say Dylan tested negative and I could come be by his side. In another odd COVID rule, I did **not** to have to be tested to enter the ER. How does that make sense? There was never any consistency. I was stressed, worried, and tired. Luckily for me, the nice security person must have noticed the dazed look in my eyes as he gave me directions to Dylan's room, because he stopped talking and just told me to follow him.

When I got inside the ER, I was surprised to find that this hospital did not separate COVID patients by floor like every other hospital I had been in. Some ER rooms were taped off with plastic walls and had a COVID sign, while others were not. The rooms seemed intermixed, with no real pattern to them. Is it even safe for Dylan to be here?

When I got into Dylan's room, the doctor came in right after me and she didn't have good news. Dylan had a small bleed on his brain **and** had blood clots in his lungs. It was devastating news, it felt like life is just a continuous stream of catastrophic news. I mean, he was in the hospital for an EEG today and he has been under a doctor's care for more than seven months. How can this possibly happen? The doctor said Dylan was in such serious shape that Mercy Hospital could not handle his needs. Dylan required an ICU with specialty doctors and specific equipment, so I was thinking maybe UC Davis again. And here comes the next blow—right now, all area hospitals are full due to COVID patients and not taking new patients. Mercy Hospital was calling around looking for a hospital that could help Dylan. There was nothing they could do here, nothing anyone could do to help Dylan until someone found a hospital to take him. I never in my life imagined this could be a real problem. We live in the United States, for crying out loud! I live in a very populated area. How could there be no medical help for an eighteen-year-old boy in distress? As usual, there was nothing I could do but sit by his side and pray. Mercifully, it was only about twenty minutes later when the doctor came in and told me that Kaiser Hospital-Vacaville accepted Dylan. Vacaville was another forty-five minutes to an hour away. We waited about twenty more minutes until Dylan was taken away in another ambulance on his way to Vacaville. For at least the third time in the past seven months, I had to give Dylan a goodbye kiss not knowing if I would see him alive again.

Once Dylan left, I drove home and exchanged the wheelchair van for my truck. Sadly, I knew I wouldn't need the van again for a while. I knew he was going to be in the hospital for an extended stay again. It was now one a.m. but the entire family was awake, including my mother in Pennsylvania where it was four a.m. I spoke with her as I drove the forty-five minutes to Vacaville. I was all out of the meds I had been given to help with my emotions, and I was crying as I got into my truck, but I made myself a promise that I would calm down. I didn't want to upset my mom any more than she already was. It was time to be strong and positive and remove the negative thoughts. I had to do this for my mom, for Dylan, and for myself. Thankfully, I was able to compose myself and I spoke to my mom without being overly emotional. She and I spoke about all good outcomes that would come from this.

I finally arrived at Kaiser Hospital-Vacaville, but when I tried to enter the ER, a security guard told me I was not allowed to enter the hospital due to COVID. I was so over COVID making everything so difficult, I felt ready to explode. Miraculously, I didn't. I kept my calm and demanded to speak with whomever was in charge. ER security had me drive around the building to the main entrance where another security guard, again, told me I could not enter. I insisted on speaking with a supervisor and when I finally got to a supervisor, I used some language Matthew had armed me with: "My disabled child is non-communicative, and I am his caregiver. I must be with him for him to receive proper medical treatment." It worked; now I was armed with a way to defeat the COVID lockdown bullshit quickly. I just needed to get to a supervisor and cite my rights as a caregiver when I was turned away. Instead of begging on their emotions, I would let the hospital staff know that I know I have a legal right to be by my son's side and no arbitrary COVID rule can prevent it. They made me sit in the downstairs lobby another thirty minutes because Dylan had skipped the ER and was taken right to the ICU where the doctors were assessing him. I sat in the lobby and the local police came and removed a homeless man who was trying to sleep in the lobby. I heard them offer him a ride to a shelter. It struck me how weird of a time we were living in. My world was like a Hollywood disaster movie.

Eventually, I got to Dylan's room, and they told me he had stabilized. COVID visitation rules for Kaiser Hospital-Vacaville were one person, per day, for one hour. Again, someone randomly made up that was the way to beat COVID. The nurses were all very nice to me and said they would let me stay by Dylan's side the rest of the night. They warned me that when administration staff realized I was in the room, they would likely remove me. I giggled and told the nurses, "Let them try!" It was three a.m. until I got in to see Dylan. Amazingly, he was awake, and he tracked me with his eyes as I walked across the room. The nurses suggested I leave by 6:30 a.m. so the shift bosses wouldn't realize I was there, and Cindy could come in later as Dylan's "one visitor for the day." I decided to go with that plan and Cindy got in to see Dylan around 8:30 a.m. Dylan had had a new CT scan of his brain and there were no signs of new bleeding. The decision was made to start Dylan on blood thinners to try to help the blood clots. It was a dangerous balance of thinning Dylan's blood without causing his brain to bleed more.

Cindy said Dylan was ok that day and she was told he was in no immediate danger of dying, so we decided to leave Dylan alone for the night. They had found more blood clots in Dylan's legs, and he had begun to run a low fever, but he was in the ICU, and they were treating him. Cindy left Dylan's side that night and I got into the hospital around 8:15 a.m. the next day. Just in time for BAM! Yet another big punch in the face.

As I walked in, they were wheeling Dylan out for an emergency CT scan of his head and chest. Dylan's blood pressure was dangerously low again and his heart rate was dangerously high. The treatments they were giving him were not working. The news crushed me, and I basically sat in a corner and cried and prayed the entire time he was gone. When Dylan returned, the doctors followed with a horrifying decision for me to make. Dylan's blood clots had worsened to the point that they were life threatening. They wanted to try a drug on him known as a clot buster. They were confident it would help clear up clots in Dylan's lungs and legs, but there was a strong possibility the drug could also open the bleed in Dylan's brain. The blood clots could be fatal; a brain bleed would be also. They felt the clots were the biggest threat now and the CT scan showed the brain bleed had not gotten any worse. They recommended to go with the clot buster, but were very clear that it was my choice and there were no guarantees. It really wasn't a choice though, if you are telling me he **will** die from the blood clots but only **could** die from the brain bleed then there is no other choice. This was an impossible situation, and I can't believe it's come to this. This kid survived a traumatic brain injury and five surgeries, but now these damn blood clots are going to kill him.

I had to leave the room for a minute while they put in a main line IV. I cried and cried in the waiting room and then a thought came to my head. If I worry about Dylan's death, it happens 1,000 times in my mind...if I concentrate on his life, I can become the positive energy Dylan needs in the room. That mindset helped, as it was all I concentrated on. I was able to control my emotions much better. Just to be safe, I emailed my personal doctor for an emergency prescription refill of my pills to help me control my emotions. My doctor was able to call it into the pharmacy inside the Kaiser Hospital - Vacaville and I ran downstairs and filled it. It was only three pills, but it was good to have something. I took one.

They brought me back into Dylan's room and explained the process to me. They will administer the clot buster to Dylan via the IV and monitor his neurological signs every fifteen minutes. These are the same signs they were checking when he was first admitted to UC Davis Hospital. I was told we should know within the hour if the clot busters worked and how his brain bleed was doing. Obviously, the hope is that the clots dissolve and the brain doesn't bleed. That is the win-win result we need here. Walking this road has taught me the power of praying for specific things; to be intentional with my thoughts. Here, I had some very specific things to pray for. I needed the clots to be gone and I needed his brain to not bleed any further. I watched as the clot buster was administered...here we go.

I began saying the Rosary and watched Dylan's every vital sign. Dylan began shivering like he had while at UC Davis. It reminded me of when my prayers were all about stopping his shivering. I don't recall how many times I made it through the Rosary. It was at least two times, plus some other prayers like the Guardian Angel Prayer. I just sat bedside and stared at Dylan. I was waiting for some sign that the clot buster was working. About fifty minutes into the treatment, Dylan coughed, and when I say it scared the hell out of me, I am not exaggerating. I almost jumped up out of my seat. An hour passed, and Dylan seemed ok. Now, we will just wait and pray. They will run more tests over the next few hours, but the clot buster had done what it was intended to do, and Dylan was still alive. Thank you, God.

JANUARY 2, 2021 – TWO HUNDRED THIRTY-TWO DAYS SINCE THE ACCIDENT.

Dylan is tough as hell! The clot buster worked and cleared the clots from his lungs and legs. His color and vitals went back to normal rather quickly. And best of all, the follow-up CT showed his brain did not bleed at all due to the clot buster. I spoke with the treating neurologist, and he felt that since there were no more brain bleeds and the bleeding that did occur was so small, there should be no lasting ill effects from it. He could not say why the bleed occurred but added that it could even happen with a brain that has never had trauma. I was told they will not retest at all for the clots. They will just monitor his vitals.

Dylan's vital signs have improved so much, they no longer worry about the clots. Dylan will be moved out of the ICU today and will begin taking Coumadin to thin his blood. It will take a few days for the Coumadin to take effect, then he should be good to come home. How long had the blood clots been a problem? Why wasn't Dylan on blood thinners earlier? I don't know these answers. I guess it has to do with his multiple surgeries and then transferring doctors and hospitals. I believe it was missed by someone, but my energy must be on Dylan.

Maybe we should get him a bike at home so he can exercise like he used to do at Craig Hospital. It is now 2021, and we finally have some good news around Dylan. I am beginning to believe that 2020 was just a cursed year. Thank God for the New Year!

JANUARY 7, 2021 – TWO HUNDRED THIRTY-SEVEN DAYS SINCE THE ACCIDENT.

Dylan comes home from Kaiser-Vacaville today, he has been there nine days. His Coumadin levels are taking a while to get to where they need to be, so they are prescribing him Lovenox. We will have to give him injections in his stomach (love handles, really) two times per day. We have had some family debate about Dylan coming home. Some feel like Kaiser is pushing him out of the hospital. I understand that point of view from a medical standpoint. But I am leaning the other way; I think too much time in the hospital is bad for him. It is a big challenge for us to care for him, but if Dylan is ever going to get better, we are the ones who will make it happen. Being in the ICU was necessary but being in a regular room, Dylan gets very little attention and almost no therapy. He is better off with us. Six months ago, I had no real medical training. Now, I give my son injections in his stomach, feed him through a tube, suction out his saliva when necessary, and care for his bathroom needs. Life comes at you fast.

These clots and the brain bleed were a very scary situation, and we are all very nervous about caring for Dylan and possibly missing signs of trouble. It really is scary, but ironically, I don't really trust the hospitals much more than us. For starters, my mom and sister bought Dylan a Fitbit and if he is wearing it, we can see his heart rate at any moment. His increased heart rate was a sign of the blood clots, but we didn't know to look for it. We also bought an automatic blood pressure cuff so we can take Dylan's vital signs several times per day and watch for any changes. There were signs there for the blood clots, but we didn't monitor Dylan's blood pressure closely enough, nor had we any idea we needed to. The once-a-week visit, for less than an hour from a nurse, was not enough, go figure. We will be administering anti-seizure meds and Lovenox to Dylan daily. We, Dylan's family, will watch for future signs of distress while also stimulating him. Dylan has been more alert now that the blood clots have been addressed. He keeps his eyes open for longer periods of time. He is already squeezing the doctor's hands and releasing on command. How long has this really been the issue? I have no way to know, and that part is extremely frustrating.

JANUARY 11, 2021 — TWO HUNDRED FORTY-ONE DAYS SINCE THE ACCIDENT.

We had Dylan at our house for two nights this weekend and it was extremely hard. Much more stressful than I imagined. It is considerably easier to do something when you know you have back up around. At Craig Hospital, when they had me perform the tasks of caring for Dylan, they were there to answer questions or correct me if I did something wrong. Erica is always here to back me up, but we are both new to this. We just try our best and hope it is good enough. We are on our own with Dylan and it is intimidating. Much like when Dylan was first hurt, the unknown is the hardest part. For the first time, I had to give Dylan an enema and do his bowel program, alone. Craig Hospital had given me the skills, but I was on my own now. I also had to put on his condom catheter and give him his Lovenox shot for the first times by myself. The shot was by far the easiest of the three.

The stress made for some tense times between Erica and me. When I am stressed, I tend to bark orders; that's my old police training. I bark orders even if I don't know exactly what I am doing. Erica would do anything for me, or Dylan, but one thing she does not like, is to be barked at, and who can blame her? I was uncomfortable and it was showing. That said, we did it. We did everything we needed to and were better at it the second time around. Our communication was stronger due to those struggles, and our confidence was increased. This was also a very emotional time for Erica because it was her first time really experiencing firsthand how bad off Dylan really is. It is one thing to hear about Dylan being unresponsive, but the hands-on experience really drives it home. When you are the one wiping the drool from the corner of the mouth of last year's leading tackler in the Sierra Football League, it really sinks in. It takes so much to care for him. It takes two hours every night just to get him into bed and one and a half hours every morning just to get him up and ready. This is a lot, and it's terribly exhausting.

Dylan's vitals are better, and his alertness is improved also. This is the reason we are doing all of this, and it is the fuel to keep us going. We are not getting much out of him physically right now but considering he is just finally waking up, I still believe there is hope for improvement. Ty and Bella also got to spend time with Dylan up close and it is hard to handle. Bella did well and helped where she could. Ty is more withdrawn, which is his personality, but also, I know it is because Dylan was the bigger, stronger stepbrother. A football star and popular, and now he needs all this help. Adult minds have a hard time dealing with that, young minds are seeing that human vulnerability for the first time. We all deal with it in our own way. The last thing I want, or Dylan would want, would be for this to negatively impact anyone else's life moving forward.

JANUARY 22, 2021 – TWO HUNDRED FIFTY-TWO DAYS SINCE THE ACCIDENT.

Caring for Dylan is the hardest thing I have ever done, but it is 1,000 percent worth it. We have settled into the pattern of one week at my house and one week at Cindy's house. I would never wish divorce on anyone, but this pattern of one week on and one week off is great for us. I cannot imagine how it would work otherwise. Trying to balance Dylan's care with work, home, and kids is next to impossible. We are hoping to eventually get some outside help with him, but in the meantime, Erica has been amazing for me. She cares for and loves Dylan deeply. She works hard to keep everyone happy and showers Dylan with love and kisses all the time, which is not easy because at this stage, he cannot really return the love. She amazes me. I knew she was special, but no one can know how someone will react in a time of tragedy until it happens, and no one saw this coming.

FEBRUARY 2, 2021 – TWO HUNDRED SIXTY-THREE DAYS SINCE THE ACCIDENT.

This is our week with Dylan. It is still very time consuming and difficult but still totally worth it. Dylan is making small gains. He is moving his left hand more than he did last week and can put his left arm around you to give a hug. He can also hold onto the bed rail of his hospital bed when being dressed, which now makes it possible for one person to do it alone. Erica can be there for Ty and Bella while I get Dylan ready for bed. Dylan is also beginning to lean himself forward in his chair and can lean himself back in a controlled manner. He can also make the *"ahhhhh"* sound on command. This may all sound insignificant, but it is progress, finally. These are the things I saw patients doing at Craig Hospital. I've been trying to deal with the State agencies to get some help and it is frustrating and slow, but we have learned to not be easily deterred. We are doing this all on our own now. We are sad, mad, and frustrated at many things, but at the same time we give Dylan love and affection and encouragement. We are **IT** for him, and we will not let him down.

We bought small white towels to keep on Dylan's chest all day to catch his drool. Dylan still has the special attachment on his wheelchair to keep his head from tilting to the side, since his neck is not strong enough to support him. Also, Craig Hospital taught us to use a small timer that beeps every twenty minutes. When it beeps, we tilt Dylan's wheelchair back all the way to shift his weight. Hopefully this will prevent bedsores. Also, we have a special air mattress for Dylan to

PAUL AND ERICA RICHARD

sleep on, which shifts his body weight throughout the night to prevent bedsores. The mattress was lent to us by the Fritz family. It would have cost us thousands of dollars to buy on our own. There are no words to properly thank people like the Fritz family! They are now part of our family forever.

FEBRUARY 23, 2021 – TWO HUNDRED EIGHTY-FOUR DAYS SINCE THE ACCIDENT.

Time flies…it goes by fast when we have Dylan because we are so busy. It also blurs by when we don't have him, because we try to cram everything else in. Dylan is slowly improving, which makes everything more bearable. Last week we worked with Dylan on standing and now he can stand up with a medium amount of help. Imagine what he could be doing if he were at Craig Hospital now? He would finally be like the patients I saw improving all around us. We help him stand using a special belt around his waist. We get him to a sitting position on the edge of a massage table we bought, so he is closer to a standing position. He is also getting more reliable with headshakes for yes and no. He can give fist bumps and even counts a little in his head. The other day while getting him to do small exercises, I added a little difficulty. I asked him to do some simple math and Dylan did it with some success. I had him kick my hand with his foot seven times. When he was done, I told him I wanted him to make it a total of ten, and he kicked his leg four more times. I think he may not have counted one because he swung his leg but it didn't hit my hand. Either way, he is improving, and that is all that matters. God is great! The path is different now and still very slow going, but at least it is going in the right direction.

FEBRUARY 26, 2021 – TWO HUNDRED EIGHTY-SEVEN DAYS SINCE THE ACCIDENT.

The year 2021 has so far been much better than 2020, but unfortunately today we received another punch in the gut. Dylan was at Cindy's house this week and when Pablo checked on him this morning, he found Dylan having a seizure. They called the paramedics but by the time they got there, Dylan seemed fine. They said everything looked fine and left. A short time later, Dylan had two more seizures and they had to return and transport him to the hospital. Dylan had two more seizures while en route to Kaiser Hospital in Roseville. He was given a shot of our old friend, Versed, and is in the ER and resting now. All his vital signs are good.

On this same day, Erica and I learned that our offer on a house better equipped for a handicapped person was accepted and I had a job interview with a company hiring people to investigate COVID-19 related fraud. As much as Dylan dictates our everyday, life doesn't just stop. The interview was on Zoom, and I had to fight myself to stop crying just before the interview so my eyes would not be puffy. We are firm believers in everything happening for a reason and while the house news is great, the job didn't work out for me, and that was for the best. It is tough to relax and enjoy anything because we never know what is next with Dylan. We have been very happy with his progress. I hope he stays as alert as he has been so he can continue to progress. I would hate to see him have to go back on heavy sedation; that would be heartbreaking.

MARCH 5, 2021 – TWO HUNDRED NINETY-TWO DAYS SINCE THE ACCIDENT.

It has been a very good week. We made it through the seizure incident about as well as we could hope. The Versed worked to stop the seizure and while he seemed tired all week, he has not had any new seizures. Physically, he continues to improve and can now stand with little help. He moves his foot like he wants to take a step, and even transferred to his bed by standing up and turning with help. We didn't have to use the Hoyer lift, which is a huge improvement in quality of life. Dylan's swallowing is slowly improving also, as he drools less. The doctors said that if he doesn't have any more seizures, they will not be increasing his anti-seizure meds. My major concern was an increase in meds making him more drowsy. I just need to accept that part of this journey will be dealing with setbacks from time to time, this one was not fun, but it does not seem to be a major setback. Stay positive and stay focused. Now we can focus some joy on getting a new house, and making it a home for our family, even if that vision has changed.

JUNE 22, 2021 – ONE YEAR AND FORTY DAYS SINCE THE ACCIDENT.

I took a break from the journal because we have been so busy. We closed on the new house in March, and have been busy making improvements before we move in. Dylan has been doing some amazing things. Unfortunately, he has also entered a very frustrating stage where he is agitated and confused a lot of the time. He refuses to do almost everything we ask. For example, he can physically stand and transfer into bed now, but he refuses. If we could count on his cooperation, we would be able to get rid of the Hoyer lift, van, and maybe even the hospital bed. We have an important meeting tomorrow with his main doctor to see what we can do. She is going to evaluate Dylan and we are going to push her to refer Dylan to CNS. CNS is a rehab in Bakersfield, California. They are not as much of a hospital as Craig Hospital. They are more of just a rehab; Craig Hospital is both. We have heard that CNS has the expertise to help Dylan as he transitions to more of a life skills-based rehab. He is alert enough to be making great progress, but the refusing is holding him back. He can speak a little now and we have begun to feed him mostly regular food. He has come so far. We continue to fight to get him the best care possible, so he recovers as much as he can. He is just about to turn nineteen years old.

How we got Dylan to start eating solid food is another example of how his family is leading him through this. Back in May 2021, Dylan was getting in-home speech therapy one time per week. In a situation like Dylan's, the speech therapist is the one who clears him to begin eating solid food. Dylan sometimes refused to cooperate at all with his speech therapist, so progress was slow, and by May 2021, Dylan was still only cleared for ice chips. My mom came to visit us that month and one day we were all in the new house and had ordered pizza. My mom, Erica, Matthew, Gabby, and I were all around. I noticed Dylan was looking at the pizza and following it around with his eyes. I decided there were enough people there—and my mom being a nurse—that if he began to choke, we would be able to give him the Heimlich maneuver. So, I handed him a piece of pizza. Dylan's deep-seeded behaviors took over and like a real East Coast-born boy, Dylan took the piece of pizza and folded it in half before rolling his eyes as he leaned in and took his first bite of real food in over a year. He ate every bite without any issue and asked for another slice. It was amazing!

JULY 5, 2021 – ONE YEAR AND FIFTY-THREE DAYS SINCE THE ACCIDENT.

Dylan is nineteen now. We tried to take him fishing for his birthday but the lake we chose was so low due to the drought that his wheelchair could not make it to the water. We still managed to have a great time as we sat around a picnic table in the park and told Dylan stories. We really needed a relaxing day because Dylan has been so difficult. He still fights everything we ask him to do and now he even throws in a curse word, or an insult, every now and then. He is very hard to manage right now. He refuses to participate in therapies and wants to lay in bed all day long. I must remind myself how hard we prayed just to have him here with us. We need to stay positive and move forward down our road, hopefully we move through this stage.

OCTOBER 27, 2021 – ONE YEAR AND ONE HUNDRED SIXTY-FIVE DAYS SINCE THE ACCIDENT.

I took a long break from journaling and probably should not have. Journaling has helped me organize my thoughts and emotions and stay positive. Dylan completely stopped participating in the home therapies Kaiser was providing. They were only one time per week for OT, PT, and ST, which was painfully insufficient anyway. We decided to take a little break from the professional therapists. Part of me was scared this could be the end of his recovery. We were always told there would be a plateau. In addition to stopping therapies, Dylan started being outright mean to certain people. He started with Gabby and Erica, but then changed to focus his anger on his mom and his friends Lucas and Kinsey. He just openly acts like he doesn't like them. Kinsey stopped coming because of it; Lucas tries to laugh it off when he visits, but I am sure it hurts him. It hurts me to see. And poor Cindy, she has been through everything I have been through, and now she must deal with his meanness. So far, I have managed to avoid being the target of it. He typically says he prefers to be with me, although that still doesn't mean I can get him to participate in therapies. We have gotten the doctors to start him on 10 mg of Prozac to see if that helps. We have also started taking him to outpatient therapies at a Kaiser facility forty-five minutes away. In the beginning, Dylan would still simply refuse to participate. It is very frustrating to load him in the van, drive him forty-five minutes each way, and then end up leaving with him having done nothing. But what can we do but keep trying? Since Craig Hospital, ninety-nine percent of his therapies have come from his family members. He only eats solid food because we pushed him every day. We constantly encourage, and even trick him into performing PT, OT, and ST exercises, some taught to us by the therapists, and some improvised by us.

We have also recently started taking him to hyperbaric treatments. We found a chiropractor's office in Granite Bay, California, which will assist him by using the Hoyer lift to put him in the hyperbaric chamber. Of course, this is 100 percent on us, insurance would not recommend it, or help pay for it. We have had several people recommend hyperbaric treatment to us, including the family member of some personal friends, who has a very tragic story himself, after suffering multiple concussions during an NFL career. This is where we have now begun to see a rebirth of improvements for Dylan. We began to see improvements every week once we started the hyperbaric treatments. It was kind of hard to keep up. He would go to Cindy's house for a week and come back with big improvements, and he returns to Cindy's a week later doing even more. We were able to completely stop using his feeding tube and convinced the doctor to have it removed. Dylan was getting better at taking steps, so we got him a walker and he just kept getting better, and better, at using it. We began playing card games with him and while it was a little rough at first, he began recognizing the card colors and values, and began playing the games. These are all things he would have excelled at in a controlled therapy situation, but that is not how our road went. We began to see some of his longer-term deficits such as short-term memory and the random meanness to some people come out. How long will he struggle with these, where is the plateau? The truth is, no one has any idea. He also has very little impulse control, but luckily for us it manifested itself in a kind of positive way. Dylan yells to everyone he sees that he loves them. Going in and out of therapies, to and from hyperbaric, Home Depot, anywhere we take him, he yells "I love you" to everyone he sees. We learned to tell people, "He is a lover," or to say, "Three weeks ago he could not speak." Most people understand and many even responded in a positive way.

In early October, we finally convinced Kaiser that nineteen-year-old Dylan would greatly benefit from a professional in-patient rehab. They chose a Kaiser facility in Vallejo, California. We wanted Dylan to go to the CNS facility in Bakersfield because we felt they were more focused on life skills. But we will take what we can get. We got eighteen days in Kaiser-Vallejo. We decided not to fight them and just accept it. Dylan was in in-patient therapy from October 5 until October 22.

In-patient was harder than I thought it would be. Dylan physically did very well, but it was hard on the family. We stuck to our standard that someone was always there with him. If he was sleeping, we stayed in a hotel nearby, but if he was awake, we were by his side. Dylan didn't really need a hospital setting at this point; he needed therapies, and he needed people who understood his injuries. When you go to a rehab, the rehab doctors get full control of all the patient's meds. Getting a fresh set of doctors was a good thing. They immediately increased his Prozac to 20 mg per day and stopped his Coumadin, since he was moving around a lot more now, blood clots were no longer a worry.

Physically Dylan began walking, using hiking poles and some balance assistance. They also got him to start using the bathroom by himself. This was a **major** milestone and one we had no idea how to accomplish at home. It was not a simple thing to accomplish, but this step makes life closer to normal for him and relieves one of our most dreaded duties. This alone was worth bringing him to Vallejo. Dylan exhausts easily and by the last few days, he was refusing some therapies but there was marked progress. Dylan began reading small words and had some success with relaying the meanings of words. He can throw the football and likes playing games. Dylan had a psychiatrist assigned to him, but other than increasing the Prozac, she could only really offer us hope that over time, more of his behaviors may improve. She really thought it was up to time to show any real improvements in his meanness and impulse control. We are blessed by how far Dylan has come. We will wait and continue to pray for more improvements, but we are grateful for where we are.

Dylan came home from Kaiser-Vallejo with a smaller wheelchair, no need for a condom catheter, and stronger physically. I had to install grab bars in his bathroom to increase his independence and allow him to stand up on his own. He is really becoming more mobile and independent. He still takes constant supervision but now it is for different reasons, like putting things in his mouth or trying to stand on his own. Dylan seems happy, not depressed. I cannot complain about anything; he has met and exceeded my prayers already. He laughs and loves. He gives kisses and hugs. Time and his family's attention seem to be his keys. We are starting back at hyperbaric treatments, looking to sell his van, and researching getting him stem cell therapy. Stem cell therapy is something else our extended family of TBI survivors has recommended we try.

This journey has been exhausting for all of us but there is hope, and hope is what we prayed and worked so hard for all these months. Dylan's life changed forever on May 12, 2020, as did ours, but it can still be a good life for all of us. Erica has been my rock through it all. Family, football community, law enforcement community, and even total strangers have gotten us this far. My faith in God is stronger than ever and we keep walking the road! We are truly blessed and lucky!

Some people can look back on certain events in their lives and are grateful for the change in their destiny. Others can only see the destruction caused by specific circumstances that somehow altered the course of where they thought they were headed. I think I fall somewhere in between. I can find anger and pain in the events of 2020, but I also completely comprehend that God has a plan for me, my family, and especially, Dylan. Sometimes our unanswered prayers can become our greatest blessings. I have never been so ignorant to believe that I am smart enough to know what's good for me. I know that my life has a purpose and there is a reason that surpasses my understanding for why this happened to my son. Looking at Dylan now, I am so proud and in awe of his strength, and I know he is going to find his way through this tragedy to make some sort of sense of it in our lives. Of course, I wish it never happened, but I can find beauty and reasoning through the pain. I can only pray someday I'll understand. Until then, I will walk the road God has laid about before me with faith and resolve, and I'll stay strong for as long as Dylan needs me.

Epilogue

I stopped journaling as Dylan continued to recover. This journey has been long and extremely trying to this point, but well worth it. A part of me wishes I would have kept going in the journal just to add detail into the time that has passed, and the improvements Dylan continues to make. In addition to the hyperbaric chamber therapies, Dylan has undergone two stem cell therapies. We have also frozen some of his stem cells that were harvested from his own body fat in hope that future gains in the field of stem cell treatment may discover better ways to benefit him. None of that would have been possible without the generosity of those who donated to his cause. There will never be an end to this journey. This family will never stop trying to give Dylan everything he needs. Our life is different than we imagined but it is very much a life of love; we can be happy in Amsterdam.

Dylan slowly continues to make small gains, to become slightly better at certain tasks, or to recall a name or the day of the week quicker than before. Dylan loves his friends and texts and Snapchats with many of them. His impulse control issues have become apparent during these conversations, but the incredible young men and women he calls friends deal with it as part of recovery. I am sure their life with Dylan as their friend is a little different than they imagined also.

Dylan still walks with a walker for longer trips or uses a cane when he is around the house. He loses his train of thought often and gets overwhelmed if there is too much going on at once. He is a jokester and loves music so much, he is constantly singing **very** loud, pretty much all the time. Although not always on key...we celebrate these moments. Dylan has suffered small seizures on two different occasions spaced about a year apart that resulted in us needing to call 911. We will continue to wait and hope that he goes longer and longer without a seizure so we can begin to reduce his medicines. We look for therapies and situations to help Dylan grow and we have even been doing extensive research on possible educational opportunities. He has disabilities, but he can learn, and tells us he will be going to college one day. I wouldn't doubt him. He certainly seems happy at home, and we are all sure he will continue to improve. He knows how to pull off a good prank and has the best belly laugh when he gets going.

Between staying with us and staying with his mom, Dylan calls them both home and we have all made the adjustments to allow for his disabilities. He has a routine which includes staying up too late and playing video games too long. He loves his food and never misses a meal. I regularly take Dylan to a local restaurant to watch the Philadelphia Eagles play. With the time difference, we are sometimes there at ten a.m. eating breakfast and cheering them on. I have taken Dylan fishing several times. We must find easy access to places, but when we do, Dylan seems to have retained his uncanny luck with a rod and real. It's pretty cool to watch.

We continue to hear TBI stories with happy endings, oftentimes ten or more years after an accident. This wasn't a six-month injury, not even a three-year journey. This is our life now; Dylan didn't quit, and neither will we. Any proceeds from his story will go to bettering his life, maybe he can eventually live semi-independent in a small place we build him on our property. This is a thought I could not even fathom in the middle of this ride.

Our hope is that this story can help someone going through similar struggles. May it help them to keep their faith, fight for their loved one, and NEVER ever give up. We are all capable of amazing things when we have no choice; just don't quit. Keep doing the right thing, keep walking that road, even if it is just one step at a time. The adjustment to our new life in "Amsterdam" has been amazing. Before the accident, I took for granted the family photo on holidays and now I cherish every moment when we can get everyone together.

There are literally hundreds of people we would like to thank and who should be mentioned in this book. There is just no way to name them all and do them the justice they deserve for the support they brought into our lives. It is through this strength, love, and support that got us this far and keeps us going.

When family members read the early drafts of this book, they often mentioned people I failed to name, or pointed out they had no idea certain people contributed so much. I know no one helped with the intention of being thanked, but they all deserve it. The kindness of others gave us the ability to focus on Dylan when he needed us, and that was the very heart of this journey. The COVID pandemic did so many bad things to this world, but during this journey, it showed how the determination and love of family, friends, and even strangers would not be stopped and shines through, lighting the path as we walked it. I am so grateful for the things that occurred during this incredible trial, but looking back, it's hard to think how I would change it. Of course, I would remove the pain and anguish, but the things I learned and have been taught throughout are difficult to reconsider. Maybe I just wasn't as "well-traveled" as I thought. The world is certainly full of beautiful places…if I can only open my mind.